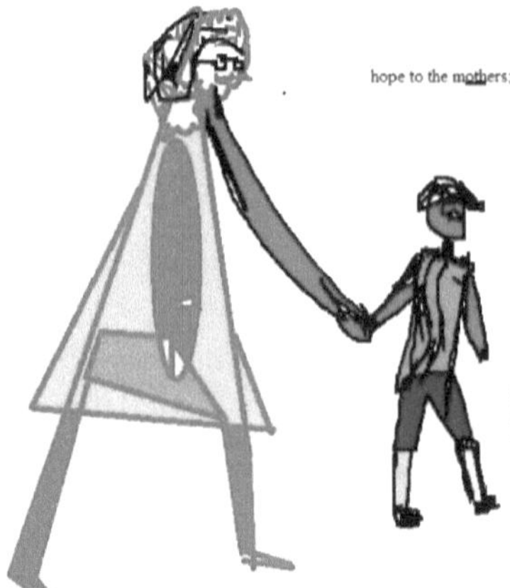

SCOLIOSIS

HOW TO PREVENT AND TREAT SCOLIOSIS
WITH THE SPINAL ACTIVE FLEXION EXERCISES
(S.A.F.E.)

NEW CLASSIFICATION OF IDIOPATHIC SCOLIOSIS AND
HOME EXERCISES TO PREVENT AND TREAT SCOLIOSIS IN
THE PRIVACY OF YOUR HOME IN YOUR OWN BED

NO NEED TO GO TO THE GYM OR EXPENSIVE
EQUIPMENTS TO BUY

BY S.ELIA

SCOLIOSIS

HOW TO PREVENT AND TREAT SCOLIOSIS WITH THE SPINAL ACTIVE   FLEXION EXERCISES (S.A.F.E.)

NEW CLASSIFICATION OF IDIOPATHIC SCOLIOSIS AND HOME EXERCISES DONE IN THE PRIVACY

OF YOUR HOME IN YOUR OWN BED
,WITHOUT ANY EQUIPMENT.

S.ELIA

SCOLIOSIS

A FRESH LOOK AT WHAT CAUSES
THE IDIOPATHIC FUNCTIONAL
SCOLIOSIS AND HOME EXERCISES
TO   STOP THE PROGRESSION OF
THE CURVE AND EVEN REVERSE
IT BACK TO NORMAL

 HOPE TO EVERY MOTHERS
ANGUISH FOR HER CHILDS
CROOKED SPINE

TRYING TO TAME THE ABNORMAL DANGEROUS CURVES WITH HOME EXERCISES FOR ALL THOSE WHO ARE DIAGNOSED WITH SCOLIOSIS, TO STOP THE PROGRESSION OF THE ABNORMAL SPINAL CURVE AND GET A HEALTHY, FLEXIBLE STRONG SPINE.

 Scoliosis is the million dollar question? How to prevent   it and how to stop the progression of the abnormal spinal curve with home exercises! And the answer is THE SPINAL ACTIVE FLEXION. EXERCISES!!(S.A.F.E.)

Disclaimer:

This book is for information ONLY
and is not intended to serve as
medical advice. Anyone seeking
specific advice or assistance should
consult his or her doctor. If they do
not like the advice of their doctor they
should seek a second opinion from
another doctor.

THE AUTHOR

S.ELIA

DEDICATION:

I Dedicate this book to all those people that will do my designed spinal active flexion exercises(S.A.F.E.) daily and get a strong, healthy, flexible spine and stop the progression of their abnormal spinal curve, the so called IDIOPATHIC SCOLIOSIS and even reverse it, and above all have a healthier life.

 It is also dedicated to all those mothers that worry about their kid's health when they are first diagnosed with scoliosis and by encouraging

their youngsters to do   THE S.A.F.E.
exercises daily, will give them hope
and eliminate their anguish and
frustration when they see their kids
getting better and have a healthy,
strong and flexible spine

THE AUTHOR

S.ELIA

TABLE OF CONTENTS

CHAPTER ONE

PROLOGUE

I write this book mainly for all the mothers and their youngsters that are first diagnosed with scoliosis and were told" to wait and see how the abnormal spinal curve, the scoliosis, will develop in six months, a year Etc..." The wait and see approach is not good enough and most of the time we know what will happen, the scoliosis gets worse. Instead they should stop whatever is causing their abnormal curve and start corrective exercises to stop the progression of the scoliosis and even reverse it back to its normal straight position.

There are many books about scoliosis which describe what scoliosis is and what the available treatments are. However all authors describe the scoliosis as idiopathic, that there is no known cause of the abnormal spinal curve and that there is nothing to do about it when is diagnosed until it is time to use braces and finally have surgery to stabilize the spine with rods and spinal fusion. I am sure the doctors do the best they can with

what they know and they do a good
job in stabilizing the spine with rods
and fusion however the patients lost
the normal function of the spine.

 For years , I and a lot of other
people, were convinced that scoliosis
was due to poor posture, slouching ,
and bad sitting habits, and still
think they cause scoliosis and other
health risks.

The so called Idiopathic scoliosis
occur during the growing years of the
kids, it affects about 2-3% of the
youngsters and affects more the girls
than the boys and that made me
thinking why is that? For years I was
wondering why more girls had
scoliosis than the boys, until   One
day while watching kids play in the
neighborhood park, I had the AHA
MOMENT .

Young kids mostly girls were lifting
other younger kids and holding them
on one side of their bodies and
carrying them around . So I figured
out that if kids do this on a daily basis
with their younger siblings, cousins,
nephews etc that's HOW   most of the
kids   get their scoliosis. So I renamed

the idiopathic scoliosis in youngsters
"THE KIDS LIFTING BABIES
SCOLIOSIS " OR BABYSITTING
JUVENILE SCOLIOSIS" When they
baby-sit, PLAY or take care of
babies.

The answer might be simple and the
idiopathic scoliosis is not idiopathic
anymore but it is a serious cause that
nobody paid any attention to it before.
Who could think that the idiopathic
scoliosis is caused with kids lifting
other kids while playing and having
fun? We give girls dolls to play with
and when they are older they like to
play with LIVE HEAVY babies, sibling,
nieces, nephews or the neighbors'
babies. sometimes babies might be
very heavy and if they have access to
these kids daily for a long period of
time AND THEY LIFT THEM AND
CARRYING THEM AROUND ON ONE
SIDE OF THEIR BODIES that's where
their scoliosis start...............
BINGO!!!!!

That's why girls have scoliosis more
than the boys.

The motherhood instinct.

CHAPTER TWO

WHAT IS SCOLIOSIS

SCOLIOSIS IS A SPINAL DISORDER
THAT CAUSES AN ABNORMAL
CURVE OF THE SPINE TO THE SIDE
,AFFECTS ABOUT 2-3% OF THE
POPULATION CAN OCCUR AT ANY
AGE BUT MOSTLY   BETWEEN THE
AGES OF 8 AND 20 and affects
MORE girls than boys.
The spine or as otherwise known THE
VERTEBRAL COLUMN has a total of
33 vertebrae ,7 in the cervical region
,that's the neck bones, 12 vertebrae
in the thoracic region, 5 in the
lumbar region , that's the low back, 5
sacral vertebrae which are fused
together and they form the base of the
spine, and 4 coccygeal vertebrae
which are also fused together . The

spine with the 24 vertebrae from the sacrum to the base of the skull forms a hollow canal which encloses and protects THE SPINAL CORD which is an extension of the brain... From the spinal cord arise the spinal nerves and the nerves leave the spinal canal through a small opening called the inter vertebral foramen, a total of 31 pairs of spinal nerves which supply nerve energy to all parts of the body.   .The abnormal curve called Scoliosis changes the size of the inter vertebral foramen , the opening from which the spinal nerves arise from the spinal cord, and puts pressure on the spinal cord and nerves causing pain and interruption to the nerve supply of the affected nerves..
Scoliosis   affects the skeletal system the spine, ribs, and pelvis and it also affects the brain ,central nervous system that is housed in the spinal canal , and the body's hormonal system and can damage major organs including the heart and lungs In other words the abnormal curve   called SCOLIOSIS affects the functions of the whole body .

 SCOLIOSIS IS CLASSIFIED EITHER AS STRUCTURAL IN WHICH THE

CURVE IS FIXED OR FUNCTIONAL IN WHICH THE   BONES OF THE SPINE ARE NORMAL. BOTH STRUCTURAL AND FUNCTIONAL SCOLIOSIS IS TRYING TO STRAIGHTEN WHEN BENDING FORWARD. (ADAM 'S TEST)

The abnormal curve of the spine is usually   S or C in shape and it can be mild or severe. Mild scoliosis does not cause problems but if untreated leads to severe scoliosis causing aesthetic and serious health problems   .

The normal human spine is straight when you see it from the back or the front but the spine   with scoliosis has abnormal curvatures to the side .

When you x-ray the scoliosis spine you will see   a sideways curve which can be measure with the COBB angle method and can vary from a mild a few degrees up to many degrees.
 The bigger the COBB ANGLE the worse the scoliosis is.

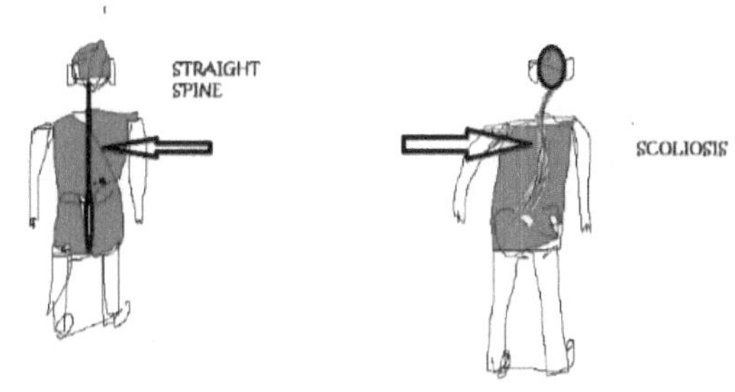

Scoliotic   spines are seen only in humans and very rarely in animals.

CHAPTER THREE

HISTORY OF SCOLIOSIS

The ancient Greeks had a saying "A HEALTHY MIND IN A HEALTHY BODY". They recognized the importance of a healthy strong body and they were spending hours to exercise to have a good strong body. They organize the Olympics and other regional games every year to show off their achievement in the development of physical abilities. They were training their youths to be both physical and mentally strong.

Despite all their efforts there were some cases of scoliosis due to injuries or some pathology and Hippocrates the father of medicine was the first to recognize and describe the condition. He devised some contraptions to treat the scoliosis with some of his ideas are still used to-day by some trying to straighten the abnormal curve.

The Spartans in ancient Greece
had the best trained soldiers of that
era, and hey started the training of
their soldiers at age 7.Their daily
routine was to swim in the river
Eurotas, strenuous exercises in the
art of fighting and other exercises.
The body of these youngsters was
strong and flexible and they had no
scoliosis or other spinal problems.
This might be an indication that with
daily exercises, swimming and other
exercises, keeps the spine healthy,
strong, and can prevent scoliosis.

From the ancient time of Hippocrates
the father of medicine till now, people
tried to correct the abnormal
curvature of the spine called
SCOLIOSIS. UNFORTUNATELY they
have not invented any magic pill YET
to correct the abnormal curvature of
the spine.

They managed to find the cause of
scoliosis from infections such as polio
and tuberculosis and other
pathological conditions, and by
treating properly those diseases they
manage to eliminate the scoliosis that
were caused by those diseases. They
had success in eliminating

poliomyelitis and treat tuberculosis that were causing pathological scoliosis but other forms of scoliosis are still a mystery and researchers are searching to find the cause of scoliosis.

 So far they did not come up with a cause and they simply call it idiopathic scoliosis, which means they do not know the cause.

Every year governments and other organizations spend millions of dollars in research to find the cause and treatment of scoliosis. The real question is, have they been looking at the right place? I.e. The youngsters that are affected with scoliosis and their lifestyle habits and environment?

They tried hard devising braces and expensive treatments but still the quest remains. Surgery with the insertion of still rods has some success to correct it but the patients lost the normal function of the spine and there are many risks associated with any surgery.

Despite the advancement of modern medicine, in the scientific community

the cause of scoliosis remain a
mystery and they have not found a
way to prevent or a cure that is
reliable, risk free for the patients.

They fail to correct the scoliosis
because they did not know the cause
or how the scoliosis starts and if you
do not know the cause of a disease
you can not treat it successfully.
That's why they called it idiopathic, of
unknown cause. First you have to
find the cause of the disease
eliminates the cause and the patient
will get well, and of course you have to
have the full co-operation of the
patient.

CHAPTER FOUR

  POSSIBLE CAUSES OF SCOLIOSIS
AND SUGGESTED NEW NAMES FOR
THE NOW KNOWN IDIOPATHIC
SCOLIOSIS

The cause of scoliosis. Let's examine
the possible cause of the abnormal
sideways curve of the spine called
scoliosis or simply "crooked spine."

 Scoliosis has many causes:

 1) It can be due to severe trauma
and this is a medical emergency and it

is treated in hospitals by the specialist
and it is not going to be discussed
here

.2) Due to some pathology, tumors,
collapse discs, osteoporosis etc. it is
best treated by the medical specialists
and is not going to be discussed here.

 3) The IDIOPATHIC SCOLIOSIS
Which STARTS SLOWLY and
progresses with time. It is called
idiopathic because they do not know
what is causing it. This is the most
common scoliosis affecting the spine
of million of youngsters age 7 to 18 ,
the growing years and some of them
will end up having major surgeries to
correct their spines and loose their
spinal flexibility.

There are many types of scoliosis
depending on the age of the individual
but we are going to talk about the
idiopathic scoliosis that occurs to
babies the so called INFANTILE
IDIOPATHIC SCOLIOSIS which affect
babies 0-3 years of age, AND
ADOLESCENT IDIOPATHIC
SCOLIOSIS which affects youngsters
age 8 to 18. Here were are going to

examine the possible causes of this so called idiopathic scoliosis, examine ways to prevent it and with home exercises to stop the progression of the abnormal curve and even correct it when it is in the early stages , provided the patients will follow the instructions to stop doing what is causing their scoliosis and do the exercises religiously daily for ever or at least when they are adults.

   THE CAUSE OF INFANTILE idiopathic scoliosis which occurs from 0-3 years of age. Most of the authors on the infantile scoliosis they classified it as idiopathic with unknown   cause.

 However I have a different opinion and I strongly believe that infantile scoliosis has a definite cause and that's the way they position the baby while sleeping, sitting or they hold the baby. If the baby was born normal and after a while a scoliosis appears on the baby, if the baby had no falls or other unforeseen accident, then the cause of the scoliosis is due to the way they have the baby to sleep. If the baby sleeps on the stomach, or always on one side, will have scoliosis in the neck region and low back AND EVEN some face and skull malformation. The baby's skull is very soft after birth and it can easily malformed if the baby sleeps in one position for long periods of time. If the mother or the care givers carry the baby on one side of their body ALL THE TIME, the baby will have a C type scoliosis. The mother might also develop some scoliosis or pains and aches in her spine. Because I think the cause of the infantile scoliosis is due to the positioning of the baby by the care givers

 I give this type of idiopathic scoliosis a new name

POSITIONAL INFANTILE SCOLIOSIS

 to be distinguished from other forms of infantile scoliosis such as traumatic, or due to some other recognizable cause, infections, or pathology etc.

When we give this type of scoliosis a name POSITIONAL INFANTILE SCOLIOSIS, with a known cause, the BAD POSITIONS they put the baby, instead of idiopathic scoliosis of unknown cause, every one will know how to treat the condition the right way: Remove the cause that causes the scoliosis, the BAD POSITIONING.

 If the POSITIONAL INFANTILE SCOLIOSIS is recognized early by the parents and the pediatrician that looks after the baby and give the mother the right instructions the infantile positional scoliosis will reverse to a normal spine. If the pediatrician gives the mother "the regular wait and see what happens approach "and they continue the same old routine with bad positions, the baby will have spinal and health problems later on. The scoliosis will get worse with time might even need corrective surgery.

The correct instructions should be, to reverse the old position they were positioning the baby. If the baby was sleeping on his stomach, now should be sleeping on his back, and if the baby was sleeping always on the right side now should be sleeping on his left side until the spine, skull and the face return to normal. Later on when the baby starts to crawl they should

encourage the baby to crawl as much
as possible, as crawling tends to
correct the spine and that's why
animals that walk on their four feet
they do not get scoliosis.
If you get the baby some swimming
lessons   that will help a lot.

 Adolescent IDIOPATHIC SCOLIOSIS
which is the most common scoliosis
affecting youngsters 8 to 18 years of
age is called idiopathic because they
did not figured out what the cause is
YET............... I happened to believe
that adolescent idiopathic scoliosis
has a few recognizable causes which
has to do with the lifestyle of the
youngsters and possible micro trauma
which was not diagnosed properly.

If the positional infantile scoliosis (the
so called infantile idiopathic scoliosis)
is not recognized early and treated
properly the abnormal spinal curve
(scoliosis) will continue to get worse
over the years and by the time the
kids reach their teens might need
surgical intervention to stabilize   the
spine. When the scoliosis starts after
the age of 7 the cause is due to bad
posture, slouching while playing video
games and television watching and

sitting in a crooked way to read and write at home and school carrying heavy backs on one side of their body over a period of long time and straining and micro trauma in the pelvis sacrum spinal joints.

 Most of the scoliosis starts in the low back area at the lumbar sacral bones.
 I remember one of my classmates who was sitting on the desk in front of me and he had the bad habit to lean forward put his left elbow on the desk and bend his body to the left close to the book he was reading or writing and he eventually got a crooked spine (mild scoliosis) to the left.

 I am sure that many kids that have such bad habits will develop scoliosis eventually. if the doctor that first diagnoses this type of scoliosis advises the child and the parents " TO WAIT AND SEE WHAT HAPPENS APPROACH " and the child continues his bad sitting habits, his spine will get worse and eventually might need surgery to correct the scoliosis. I rename this type of idiopathic scoliosis to BAD HABITS POSTURAL SCOLIOSIS, OR JUST POSTURAL

SCOLIOSIS, because its cause is the bad posture habits and   when they do it day in day out they will develop a crooked spine. In the early stages this type of scoliosis is reversible provided that the kids stop the bad posture slouching habits and do the right exercises which I will describe under exercises   for the treatments of scoliosis.

 And finally the MYSTERY of scoliosis that affect more girls than boys it is caused when the young girls baby sit or play for long periods of time with babies, siblings, cousins nephews neighbors kids , lifting them and holding them in their arms either on left or right side .It is usually starting slowly but if they continue to do this for a long period of time the scoliosis will get worse,.

 I name this type of scoliosis BABYSITTING JUVENILE SCOLIOSIS (playing, lifting, babysitting and taking care Of younger kids).

 The doctor should ask specific questions when the scoliosis diagnosis is made to find the real cause of this not so unusual type of scoliosis.

Simply ask them if they have access to babies, siblings, nephews, cousins or other kids and if they baby-sit, play and spend long hours holding the babies.

The rest of the idiopathic scoliosis in that age group is probably caused by micro trauma, sprain or strain in their spine or the pelvis, sacrum ,spine , which was not diagnosed to be treated properly, as the youngsters might have not complained.

Just think about for a moment : how many times kids and adults slip and fall on their buttock   while walking or playing , they get some pain in their low back , but they fail to see a doctor for diagnosis and treatment if necessary. This might be the beginning of   some type of scoliosis, mild or severe if not recognized and treated properly.

When there is a strain or sprain in the lower back and pelvic joints it might create a false short leg on one side and this in return if not treated properly will cause mild spinal curve in the lower back and eventually while the body tries to straighten out

creates a new curve in the thoracic
region and that's the making of
abnormal   S CURVE Type of
scoliosis.

This type of scoliosis I will name it as

TRAUMATIC COMPENSATORY
SCOLIOSIS

 due to a false short leg, and my
guess is that's the cause of the
majority of the so called idiopathic
scoliosis.

If you examine these patients while
lying face down you will notice that
they have an apparent short leg and
if you ask them they probably tell you
that they did have a fall , strain or low
back pain which they did not seek
treatment.......if not they might have
a true short leg that is causing their
scoliosis and you have   to fix that
with a shoe lift on that side in order
to have any success in treating their
scoliosis. If a true short leg is
causing S type of scoliosis I name
this as:

 SHORT LEG COMPENSATORY
SCOLIOSIS.

Now that we know what causes each type of scoliosis, instead of calling it IDIOPATHIC, we will try to eliminate the cause   and with the full cooperation of the patients their scoliosis should improve or even reverse . Without the patients cooperation no treatment can be successfully.

We took the so called IDIOPATHIC SCOLIOSIS,   with no known cause, we examined the possible causes and re-classify it according to its cause with a known OR possible cause. And I have reclassified to:

1)POSITIONAL INFANTILE SCOLIOSIS (from the old infantile idiopathic scoliosis which is caused when the mother or care giver hold the babies on one side or place the babies in one side when they sleep.)

2)BAD HABITS POSTURAL ADOLESCENT SCOLIOSIS OR JUST POSTURAL ADOLESCENT SCOLIOSIS (from the old idiopathic adolescent scoliosis ,which is caused by bad postural habits in their daily lives.)

 3)BABYSITTING SCOLIOSIS (from the old juvenile idiopathic scoliosis that affect more girls than boys and the cause is babysitting or lifting and playing with babies)

 4)TRAUMATIC COMPENSATORY SCOLIOSIS (from the old idiopathic juvenile scoliosis)this type of scoliosis is due to untreated strains, sprains, or other injuries to the low back and pelvic joints. or by just kids being kids fooling around or playing practical jokes or even bending down to pick their ball and can get a low back strain .)

 5)SHORT LEG COMPENSATORY SCOLIOSIS (From the old idiopathic juvenile scoliosis, when there is a true short leg .)

 In conclusion There is always a Cause of scoliosis.

There is no such thing as idiopathic scoliosis, there is always a cause from the time of birth to adulthood ..
 If the babies are born naturally with no human intervention or instrumentation they have a normal spine. The danger of developing a scoliosis spine starts right after birth with the way the parents or other caregivers will care for the child.

ONCE THE SCOLIOTIC CURVATURE STARTS TO DEVELOP IT WILL CONTINUE TO GET WORSE UNLESS THERE IS   an intervention to find out what's causing the abnormal curvature.

They should examine all possible cause from an injury from lifting or carrying something heavy to slouching. The patient should be instructed how to sit properly, sit straight, stand tall, avoid lifting heavy objects and bad posture, avoid sitting in a crooked position watching TV for long time.

CHAPTER FIVE

SIGNS AND SYMPTOMS OF SCOLIOSIS

People with scoliosis might have pain in the low back, neck and shoulder blades and sometimes in the early stages, the scoliosis can be without pain.

When the scoliosis is severe with the spine severely crooked it can cause serious health problems affecting the lungs, heart and other the parts of the body .

People with scoliosis have uneven shoulders, one shoulder blade is more prominent than the other, and have a rib hump One hip higher than the other uneven hips arms or leg lengths.

 Sometimes   other people, family friends and classmates notice the scoliosis first

CHAPTER SIX

DIAGNOSIS OF SCOLIOSIS

<u>AND SUGGESTED NEW NAMES FOR
THE NOW KNOWN   " IDIOPATHIC
SCOLIOSIS"</u>

 Anybody can see a crooked spine
when the abnormal curve is severe ,
but a   definite diagnosis is made by
taking a full x ray   of the spine with
the patient standing, AP   and lateral
views and measuring the COBB
angle to see how bad the abnormal
curve is.
The greater the   COBB angle the
worse the scoliosis is.

There is also a simple test the"
ADAMS TEST" by asking the patient
to bend forward with the knees
straight to see if there is an
abnormality on   one side of the
spine(the curve of the scoliosis) a rib
hump   where the ribs on one side
protrude.

To diagnose
the positional infantile scoliosis ,

is done by physical examination of
the baby's spine and face and if
there are indications of an abnormal
spinal curve to take x rays to confirm
the diagnosis. You will also have to
do detective work and   ask specific
questions of the mother or others who
care for the baby to differentiate   if it
is positional or has other cause such
as trauma during delivery with
instrumentation ,
a fall   at home or even some
underlying pathology or negligence.
These are the questions to ask the
mother or caregivers..

1) was the delivery normal without
instrumentations? In a difficult
delivery with the use of instruments
there is a possibility for the baby to
sustain injuries to his neck , head
and spine and cause the
scoliosis(traumatic infantile scoliosis),
wry neck, even   cerebral palsy..

2) what's the position the baby
usually sleep? a)face up on his back
b) right side all the time   c)left side all
the time d) not the same position e)
face down with the neck twisted to
one side. different positions can cause
different changes

3)is the baby sleeping well or does he wake up and cry often? (Waking up and crying might be an indication that the position the baby   sleeps causes some strain and pain)

4) any changes to his face and skull appearance since birth? When was the first time noticed the skull and face changes? any pictures of the baby at different intervals to notice any face abnormalities. pictures will show if there is a change from the time of birth. Change to the babies face is indicative that the baby sleep one side all the time or face down.

5) any accidental fall of the baby? if yes was the baby examined by a doctor? what did he say? Falls can cause injuries to the baby's spine

6)are there any siblings or other kids that hold and play with the baby? if yes how often? kids might have accidentally dropped or injured the baby.

7)did the baby had a serious
infection or serious illness that
required hospitalization for a long
time? If the child had an illness
might have effected his spine.

 8)who cares for the baby? The mother
or somebody else? Very important to
know, if someone else is caring for the
baby , might be abuse and
negligence.

From the answers you get, you will
have an idea if it is POSITIONAL
INFANTILE SCOLIOSIS, where the
baby sleeps on same side all time or
has other cause such as a fall,
negligence   or from other cause.

 To diagnose the

BAD HABITS POSTURAL SCOLIOSIS

 you have to take x-rays AP and
lateral to identify the abnormal curve
and do detective work about their
lifestyle and postural habits .
You have to have a detailed case
history and the lifestyle of the
youngster, how they sleep, how the sit
at school, at home and when they
watch television or play video games,

if they exercise , how often and what
sports they play.
 If they have bad sitting habits , sleep
face down, play no sports and do not
exercise and had no history of injury,
then it is   BAD HABITS POSTURAL
SCOLIOSIS or simply POSTURAL
SCOLIOSIS. Usually the bad habits
postural scoliosis is C TYPE
SCOLIOSIS.

THE BABYSITTING FUNCTIONAL
SCOLIOSIS

  is diagnosed from the case history
and x-rays. The x-rays confirm the
crooked spine and the case history
will differentiate it from any other
scoliosis. .The youngsters with this
type of scoliosis will have access to
babies either babysitting or playing
with them for long periods of time
lifting them holding them etc.
This type of scoliosis it can be either
C type or S Type scoliosis .They might
have strain or sprain in the low back
, sacroiliac joints from lifting the
babies   CAUSING AN ABNORMAL
CURVE in the low back and a
compensatory curve in the thoracic
region from holding the babies .or just
C curve from holding the babies on

one side of their bodies. Even boys can get this type of scoliosis when they have access to babies and they lift, or hold babies.

 The definite diagnosis of any abnormal curvature is made by x-rays and then you have to do detective work to differentiate and find the real cause.

 **The above causes that cause scoliosis mentioned are the most common causes of the so called idiopathic   juvenile scoliosis , but I am sure there are a lot more causes of scoliosis, such as unreported and untreated injuries from horsing around, playing practical jokes or injuries from playing certain contact sports such as football, soccer , wrestling and even injuries from playing on a trampoline etc. it might be very difficult to find the cause that causes scoliosis in such cases especially
if the youngsters do not remember such injuries. In such cases the term IDIOPATHIC SCOLIOSIS might be justified, until the real or possible cause is recognized .**

there is always a cause but the youngsters do no remember and did not report it .

4) to diagnose the
TRAUMATIC COMPENSATORY
JUVENILE SCOLIOSIS
   you have to do detective work to see if the patient remembers and had an untreated injury .

To confirm the diagnosis you take x-rays to see that the curve starts at the lumbar sacral area and one ileum is higher than the other causing a functional false short leg. And when you press on the pelvic joints and low lumbar joints you might elicit   pain.
You   also have to measure the leg length to make sure that is not a true short leg.

5)The   SHORT LEG
COMPENSATORY SCOLIOSIS
 is diagnosed by taking x rays to verify the abnormal curve of scoliosis and the pelvis to be lower on one side and the hip lower than

the other one. When you measure
the leg lengths' you will find that
one leg is shorter than the other. A
true short leg.

CHAPTER SEVEN

<u>SUGGESTED TREATMENTS OF</u>
<u>SCOLIOSIS</u>

  There are many treatments for
scoliosis. Some of them are good
some of them so-so and some risky
and dangerous, like the corrective
surgery and the use of rods,

although I must say that in many cases it is absolutely necessary and sometimes with good results . Most children when they are first diagnosed with a mild scoliosis they are told to wait and see how the curve will develop in six months to a year without any treatments or advice.

To   "the wait and see approach

I have to agree with Dr.. 'John H. Moe 1905-1988 a University of Minnesota orthopedic surgeon, who founded the Scoliosis Research Society in 1966 and he began a "do not delay" campaign for scoliosis, and he wrote   " procrastination was the most pernicious problem in idiopathic scoliosis and sad to see a child come with a severe curve requiring surgery with X-rays taken many years before showing a mild curve that could have been easily treated with a brace.46'Dangerous Curve" campaign

When the abnormal curve gets
worse in six months or a year they
advice them to use a brace for a
period of time and if that does not
help the scoliosis they have
surgery to fuse the spine   and use
rods to straighten the spine.

 I am not familiar with braces used
to treat scoliosis and I do not
know   what rate of success they
have   so I have no opinion
whether to use a brace or not.

 I Saw Some pictures of those
braces   and they look bulky and
uncomfortable .

 The idea of bracing probably came
from the same idea that the
farmers use straight sticks to
support their young seedling trees
so that their trunk grows straight.
It protects the young trees from
the elements of nature and works
perfectly for the young trees but
the trees do not have to go
anywhere and just stand there until
they grow and their trunk is strong
and straight.

It is a great idea for the trees but not so for the youngsters, they have to move and do things which is very uncomfortable and unable to do the usual things which   we take for granted that we should be able to do, like bending over to tie your shoes, or go to the washroom etc. plus there is pressure on certain area of their bodies ,trying to keep the spine straight and every time they move their bodies is uncomfortable and can even cause some irritation on the skin where the pressure is applied.

Anyway if some youngsters can put up with all that and do not cheat, they might see some benefits and their scoliosis will stop the progression and might even avoid the rods and spinal fusion.

Instead of bulky and heavy braces in mild scoliosis I might recommend a soft lumbar sacral support   to protect the low back from further injuries , and spinal exercises to get stronger muscles and more flexible spine . With the spinal active exercises which I designed they will also get realignment of their pelvic and hip joints to have restore normal function to those joints.

 Treatments with corrective exercises should start as soon as possible after the diagnosis of scoliosis is made to stop the progression of the abnormal curve.
  Some of the conservative treatments such as physiotherapy, the schroth method and others that have limited success may be due to the fact that they   fail to teach the patient what to avoid while getting treatments or what they should do at home.

Because if you do the exercises for 30 minutes or an hour, trying to push the spine to its normal position and the patient goes home and keeps doing what they have been doing to cause the scoliosis in the first place, it's obvious that they will put their spine to a scoliosis state AGAIN and the treatment has no effect

 For anybody who attempts to correct the scoliotic spine they must first have the full co-operation of the patient and the patient follows all the recommendations of the treating practitioner. If they do not have their full co-operation.

NO TREATMENT OR EXERCISE

will correct the abnormal curvature if f they fail to give instructions to the patient what to do after the treatment and what to avoid in between treatments ,again the treatment will not be effective or have lasting effects.

 Many of these conservative treatments are expensive and many times inconvenient as the patients have to travel long distances or they have to stay in an inpatient intensive rehabilitation program. If the patients have some correction during their stay or while getting treatments and when they go home start doing whatever they were doing to get the scoliosis in the first place, they will end up with the same old curvature or even worse.

   Since I have no idea what type of success the physiotherapy and other therapies get and I have no idea what instruction they give to their patients during and after treatments, I cannot say anything about those therapies. If the patients are satisfied with their treatment and see improvements in their condition its up to the patients to say if this or that therapy is good or not and stick with it or not.

   Besides all the known therapies including surgery , are treating the scoliosis as IDIOPATHIC   WITH UNKNOWN CAUSE , so in reality they treat the symptoms of scoliosis   and not the cause because they do not know the cause. If you do not know the cause of a disease you cannot treat it properly and remove the cause.

That's the reason why I reclassified the idiopathic scoliosis into five new names according to what is causing each type of scoliosis . .

In every type of scoliosis you have
to remove the cause first and with
the proper exercises the spinal
muscles will get stronger and have
an effect on the spinal curves
including scoliosis.

Suggested Treatments of the

INFANTILE POSITIONAL
SCOLIOSIS :

Treatments, or rather exercises
should start as soon as possible,
with the blessing of the attending
doctor, when a diagnosis is made
".The wait and see approach" is
not good enough and dangerous for
the patient.
The mother or the care giver of the
baby should switch the usual
positions that the baby was lying
sleeping or holding the baby. If
the baby was sleeping all the time
on his left side now should be
placed on his right side or on his
back. if they were holding the baby
on the right side now switch to
left. When they bathe or change

the baby they should place the baby
on his back and encourage the
baby to move his arms and legs.

 Exercises are good for everyone
including babies.

When the baby is able to crawl
encourage him to crawl as much
as possible. Encourage the babies to
sleep on their back and never face
down. when they are older give
them swimming lessons and
exercises on a monkey bar.
  It is very important to recognize
and treat the positional infantile
scoliosis early. If left unrecognized,
undiagnosed and untreated ,it will
get worse with time and might need
corrective surgeries in the future.

 And I quote from the dangerous
curve
Dr. john H .Moe 1905-1988   who
began a "do not delay" campaign
for scoliosis, and wrote "it is sad to
see a child come with a severe
curve requiring surgery with X-rays
taken many years before showing a
mild curve that could have been
easily treated with a brace."

Besides the INFANTILE
POSITIONAL SCOLIOSIS   is the
easiest to recognize and treat
successfully since it is in the early
stage and kids respond better to
treatments as they do not have to
do much, the adults that care for
the baby do all that is needed.

<u>Suggested Treatments for the bad
habits</u>

<u> POSTURAL SCOLIOSIS OR JUST
JUVENILE POSTURAL SCOLIOSIS</u>

 should start immediately as soon
as the diagnosis is made.   Remove
the cause, which are bad habits.
and emphasize that the bad habits
they have BAD affects on their
spine and unless they change their
habits the scoliosis will get worse
and they may end up having
corrective surgery with spinal
fusion and rods in their spine.

Give them instructions how to sit
when reading, writing, watch

television and how to lift properly
and of course to start the S.A.F.E.
(spinal active flexion exercises),
along with the monkey bar
exercises and swimming whenever
they have the time.

<u>The suggested treatments for</u>

<u>BABYSITTING JUVENILE</u>
<u>FUNCTIONAL SCOLIOSIS</u>

is by removing the cause which is
the association with babies, with
advising the patient to stop
babysitting, lifting or carrying
around any babies and the same
instructions as with postural
scoliosis , and the S.A.F.E.
EXERCISES , monkey bar exercises,
holding the monkey bar with both
hands and swinging back and forth ,
creating natural traction of the
spine with the weight of their body,
swimming and other sport
activities. They should start
exercising as soon as the diagnosis
is made.

" The wait and see approach is not a good option. "If they Keep babysitting and lifting heavy babies the scoliosis will get worse AND MIGHT NEED CORRECTIVE SURGERY!

The suggested treatment for

 TRAUMATIC COMPENSATORY JUVENILE SCOLIOSIS

  is more difficult to treat but by taking care of the low back by using an elastic support   for the lumbar sacral area , proper lifting instructions, good postural habits and the S.A.F.E. EXERCISES   they should see some improvement.

 The elastic support is removed when exercising.

 The monkey bar exercises and swimming should also help.

They should avoid any rough
contact sport, like wrestling,
hockey and football.

<u>The suggested treatment for the</u>

 <u>TRUE SHORT LEG JUVENILE</u>
<u>SCOLIOSIS</u>

 is treated by removing the cause
which is the short leg.

This is the type of scoliosis that
people affected with polio had
when one of their legs was affected.
They should have a heel or shoe
lift in the shoe of the affected
SHORT leg .

 With the S.AF.E.   EXERCISES ,
the monkey bar and swimming
exercises should see some
improvement in their spinal curve.

**Basically to have an improvement
in the curve of scoliosis, any type
of scoliosis, you have to remove the
cause that is causing the scoliosis,
whatever the cause is, and
EXERCISE   to strengthen the
muscles of the spine.**

Proper precautions how to
lift and good postural habits
are essential for all people
whether they have a scoliosis
or a straight spine, to protect
their spine from injury.

CHAPTER EIGHT

Reasoning for the   development and design of the   home " SPINAL ACTIVE FLEXION EXERCISES"   in short (S.A.F.E.)

Somebody said "that all the advances of the human race were made by somebody making an observation about something and somebody else adding to that observation. "

For example someone observed that wood floats on water, others added to that observation and today we have the huge ships we use.

Somebody invented the wheel and
by continually somebody adding
something to the invention of the
wheel, today we have the cars   and
everything else that has wheels.

 A   young doctor observed that the
women in a particular hospital were
dying after they gave birth in that
hospital while other women that were
having their babies delivered at home
by a midwife   were not dying, not
even getting sick.

 On further observation he noticed
that the same doctors that they were
doing autopsies on the dead mothers,
they were   examining the new
mothers to be without washing their
hands transferring the germs from
the dead mothers to the new mothers
to be and that's why the new mothers
were dying from infections.

When he asked all the doctors to
wash their hands when leaving the
autopsy room and just before entering
the room of the new mothers to be,
the deaths of the new mothers
stopped.

That's why today there is a lot of
hand washing and sterilization to
avoid infections and deaths during
medical exams and operations.

The same goes for all the other
inventions we have today that make
our lives easier.

 In 1865 William ADAMS was the first
to describe " the forward bending test
" for scoliosis, and all doctors use
this test to diagnose the functional
or structural scoliosis.

 A functional scoliosis is the one that
when the patient bends forward the
spine straightens out and it is
symmetrical at the thoracic level,
 and with the structural scoliosis
when the patient bends forward the
abnormal curvature of the spine it is
still noticeable but tries to straighten
somewhat.

 William Adams made a very good
observation about the abnormal
curve of the spine called scoliosis but
nobody added anything to that
observation or took advantage of that
observation up to now.

Based on Williams Adams
observation I designed specific
exercises for the spine so that by
bending   and exercising the spine
for long periods of time will make
the muscles of the spine stronger ,
flexible and keep it almost
straight.

Anybody who wants to correct the
scoliotic spine they must first have
the full co-operation of the patient
to do the exercises everyday
religiously , otherwise

<u>NO TREATMENT OR EXERCISE</u>

 will correct the abnormal curvature
if the patient keeps doing the bad
habits that caused the abnormal
curve in the first place.

 FOR PEOPLE THAT ARE REALLY
SERIOUS TO STOP THE
PROGRESSION OF THE ABNORMAL
SPINAL CURVE (THE SCOLIOSIS)
AND EVEN REVERSE IT BACK TO
ALMOST NORMAL

<u>THEY SHOULD DO 3 THINGS</u>

.1)STOP THE THINGS YOU ARE DOING TO CAUSE THE SCOLIOSIS, I.E. POOR POSTURE, POOR SITTING HABITS AT HOME, AT SCHOOL, PLAYING VIDEO GAMES AND SLOUCHING WHILE IN BAD SITTING POSITIONS WATCHING TELEVISION   AND CARRYING HEAVY OBJECTS BACK PACKS AND EVEN BABIES ON ONE SIDE OF YOUR BODY.

 2) SIT UPRIGHT   ON THE CHAIR AT HOME, AT SCHOOL, WATCHING TV OR ON THE COMPUTER. AND STOP LIFTING AND HOLDING BABIES. IF YOU LOVE BABIES PLAY WITH THEM ON THE FLOOR , EVEN CRAWL AROUND WITH THE BABIES AND THAT'S GOOD FOR YOUR SPINE. SIT TALL, WALK TALL , FEEL TALL AND EXERCISE. EXERCISING WILL KEEP YOU HEALTHY AND HAVE A GOOD POSTURE.

3) DO THE RIGHT EXERCISES TO STRETCH, MOBILIZE YOUR SPINE AND STRENGTHEN YOUR SPINAL MUSCLES AND THAT WILL HELP YOUR SCOLIOSIS, IT CAN EVEN REVERSE IT.

YOU HAVE TO DO ALL 3:

A) STOP THE BAD HABITS THAT ARE CAUSING SCOLIOSIS

B) GET GOOD HABITS THAT HELP YOUR SPINE STAY STRAIGHT

C) DO THE RIGHT EXERCISES S.A.F.E. I designed

RELIGIOUSLY EVERY DAY TO MAKE YOUR SPINE STRONGER, FLEXIBLE AND STOP THE PROGRESSION OF THE ABNORMAL CURVE.

IF YOU DO ONLY ONE WILL NOT HELP YOU MUCH.

I WILL DESCRIBE THE RIGHT EXERCISES

BUT YOU HAVE TO DO THE WORK FAITHFULLY DAILY,

NOBODY ELSE CAN DO IT FOR YOU.

I THINK IT IS ABOUT TIME TO RECOGNIZE THAT SCOLIOSIS IS A PREVENTABLE DISEASE AND

SHIFT THE RESPONSIBILITY TO PREVENT AND CORRECT THE ABNORMAL CURVE TO THE PATIENT   AND THEIR PARENTS,

BY GIVING   THE PATIENT THE NECESSARY TOOLS, WHICH IN THIS CASE IS THE SPINAL EXERCISES, TO DO IT, IN THE PRIVACY OF THEIR HOME IN THEIR OWN BED!

<u>NOBODY ELSE CAN DO IT FOR THEM.</u>

AND UNFORTUNATELY NOBODY WILL EVER INVENT THE MAGIC PILL TO CORRECT THE SPINAL ABNORMAL CURVES!!!

IT IS A STRUCTURAL PROBLEM AND ONLY WITH EXERCISES CAN BE PREVENTED AND TREATED SUCCESSFULLY IN THE EARLY STAGES.

IF LEFT UNTREATED AND
BECOMES   SEVERE SCOLIOSIS
THEY WILL END UP WITH
CORRECTIVE SURGERY AND RODS
IN THEIR SPINE!

FOR HOW LONG YOU HAVE TO DO
THE EXERCISES?

I SAY FOREVER OR AT LEAST
UNTIL ADULTHOOD FOR THE
GOOD OF YOUR SPINE AND YOUR
HEALTH.

THE BEST TIME TO START
EXERCISING IS YESTERDAY

BUT SINCE YESTERDAY IS GONE
START AS SOON AS POSSIBLE   OR
RIGHT AFTER THE FIRST X RAY
AND YOU WERE TOLD TO WAIT
AND SEE FOR THE NEXT X RAY.

IF YOU CONTINUE WITH YOUR OLD
BAD HABITS YOUR SCOLIOSIS
WILL GET WORSE AND MIGHT
NEED SURGERY IN THE FUTURE.

INSTEAD OF WAITING TO SEE
WHAT HAPPENS TILL THE NEXT X
RAY,

DO THESE EXERCISES AND
AVOID YOUR OLD BAD SITTING
HABITS, SIT STRAIGHT AT HOME,
AT SCHOOL AND EVERYWHERE,
DO NOT Slouch WHEN YOU WATCH
TV OR PLAY VIDEO GAMES.

 SIT TALL, WALK TALL, HAVE A
GOOD POSTURE. AND THE NEXT
TIME THEY TAKE YOUR X RAY
YOU MIGHT BE SURPRISED TO
SEE SOME IMPROVEMENT .

 THE REASON I CHOSE THESE
EXERCISES IS
 THAT EVERY SPINE WITH
SCOLIOSIS TRIES TO CORRECT
ITSELF WHEN YOU BEND
FORWARD (ADAMS TEST) SO IF
YOU BEND YOUR SPINE OVER AND
OVER ,YOUR SPINE WILL GET
STRONGER AND STRAIGHTEN
ITSELF TO A DEGREE.

WHEN I WAS DESIGNING THE
SPINAL ACTIVE EXERCISES I PUT
A LOT OF EMPHASIS ON THE
LUMBAR , SACRAL, PELVIS AND
HIP JOINTS, BECAUSE THAT'S
WHERE MOST OF THE SCOLIOSIS
START

AND BY MOBILIZING AND
CORRECTING THOSE JOINTS
WILL AFFECT THE SPINAL CURVES
ABOVE.
 YOU HAVE TO FIX THE
FOUNDATION OF THE SPINE FIRST
AND BY DOING SO THE SPINE
WILL CORRECT ITSELF.. WHEN
THE MUSCLES ARE STRONGER
AND THE   SPINAL JOINTS, HIP
AND PELVIS ARE MOBILIZED   .
OF COURSE YOU HAVE TO BE
SURE THAT THERE   NO PROBLEM
WITH THE LEG LENGTHS

 I chose not to use the standing
forward bending exercise, the
Adams test, although it is a good
exercise and will help the scoliotic
spine and I designed the exercises
to use the forward flexion of the
spine while lying down face up
taking away the gravity factor
which is present when you stand
and bend forward. Besides bending
forward while standing over and
over again might cause some strain
on the low back and might be some
other factors   that the standing
forward flexion is contraindicated,
like some abnormality in the

vertebral bones, like an undiagnosed fracture spondylolisthesis. , or spondylolysis.

 If there are no contraindications and all the vertebrae have no break in the pars interarticularis (spondylolysis) or spondylolisthesis,

 the Adam's forward bend is a good exercise to do several times a day.

  MOST OF THE EXERCISES ARE DONE

 LYING FACE UP SO THAT YOU CAN EASILY DO THE EXERCISES EVERY MORNING   RIGHT AFTER YOU WAKE UP,, NOON AND AFTERNOON WITHOUT STRAINING YOURSELF.

  ALL EXERCISES SHOULD BE DONE ON AN EMPTY STOMACH AND GO EASY AT THE BEGINNING WITHOUT STRAINING YOURSELF UNTIL YOUR SPINE GETS STRONGER AND MORE FLEXIBLE

WITH THE DAILY SPINAL
STRETCHING.

AS YOUR SPINAL MUSCLES ARE
GETTING STRONGER YOU
INCREASE THE REPETITION OF
THE EXERCISES TO HAVE BETTER
RESULTS SOONER!

CHAPTER NINE

DESCRIPTIONS OF THE HOME S.A.F.E. EXERCISES AND HERE ARE THE HOME EXERCISES WHICH I DESIGNED AND I CALL S.A.F.E. (SPINAL ACTIVE FLEXION EXERCISES)

1) spinal stretch by extending your arms above your head and your legs

extended with feet together
touching the mattress pushing
them down as much as possible

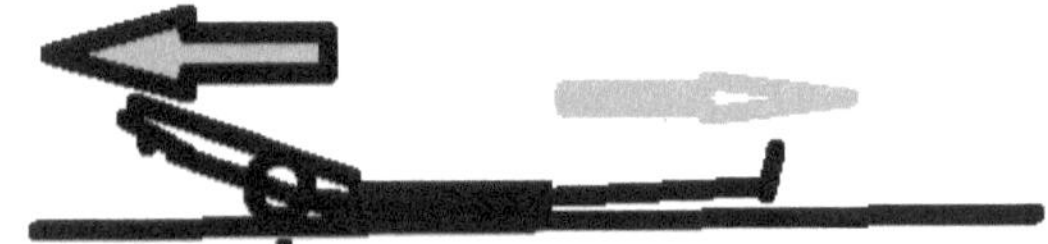

EXTEND YOUR HANDS ABOVE YOUR HEAD TRYING
TO REACH AS FAR AS YOU CAN
AND SIMULTANEOUSLY
WITH YOUR FEET   TOGETHER TOUCHING THE
MATTRESS STRETCH THEM DOWN AS FAR AS
YOU CAN

THIS IS A SPINAL STRETCH EXERCISE
FEEL THE SPINAL STRETCH

LIE FACE UP ON A FIRM
MATTRESS WITH A SMALL PILLOW
UNDER YOUR HEAD   OR YOU CAN
DO THESE EXERCISES IN YOUR
OWN BED RIGHT AFTER YOU WAKE
UP IN THE MORNING.

EXTEND   BOTH YOUR FEET
TOGETHER TOUCHING THE
MATTRESS

AND EXTEND YOUR HANDS ABOVE
YOUR HEAD AS FAR AS YOU CAN
WITH YOUR RIGHT HAND HOLDING
YOU LEFT WRIST

STRETCH YOUR HANDS UP

 AND YOUR FEET DOWN TRYING
TO EXTEND YOUR SPINE AS MUCH
AS POSSIBLE

 WHILE TAKING A DEEP BREATH
EXPANDING YOUR CHEST AS
MUCH AS POSSIBLE
 'FEEL THE STRETCH OF YOUR
SPINE

 AND HOLD IT FOR THE COUNT OF
THREE'

AND THEN EXHALE SLOWLY

REPEAT IT 5 TIMES. OR MORE

 THIS IS A STRETCHING EXERCISE
OF YOUR SPINE

 THEN EXERCISE

2) EXERCISE STRETCHING YOUR CHEST AND SHOULDER   BLADES

 LYING FACE UP WITH FEET EXTENDED

INTERLOCK YOUR FINGERS

 AND PLACE YOUR HANDS UNDER YOUR HEAD

 AND YOUR ELBOWS TOUCHING THE MATTRESS.

  THEN BRING YOUR ELBOWS TOWARDS YOUR FACE AND THEN BACK PRESSING ON THE MATTRESS.

LYING FACE UP WITH FEET EXTENDED

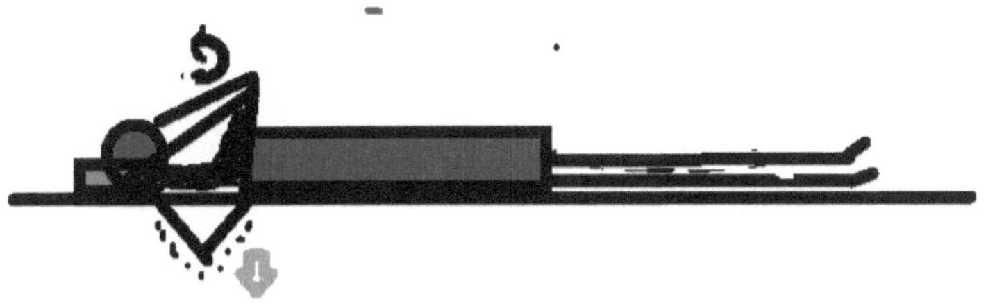

THEN
BRING YOUR ELBOWS TOWARDS YOUR FACE AND THEN BACK
PRESSING ON THE MATTRESS.

**REPEAT THIS EXERCISE 5-10
TIMES .**

**REST BY TAKING A FEW DEEP
BREATHS EXPANDING YOUR
CHEST AS MUCH AS POSSIBLE AND
THEN EXHALING SLOWLY**

**THIS IS A GOOD STRETCHING
EXERCISE FOR YOUR SHOULDER
BLADES AND UPPER BACK
MUSCLES**

THE ABOVE EXERCISES
INCREASE THE MOBILITY OF YOUR
CHEST , NECK AND UPPER BACK
STRENGTHENING THE MUSCLES
OF YOUR BACK AND SHOULDER
BLADES.

3) SPINAL STRETCH

RAISING YOUR HEAD TOWARDS
YOUR CHEST

WHILE SUPPORTING YOUR HEAD
WITH YOUR HANDS

FROM THE SAME POSITION,

LYING FACE UP ,

YOUR FEET EXTENDED

AND WITH YOUR INTERLOCKED
FINGERS SUPPORTING YOUR
HEAD,

RAISE YOUR HEAD TOWARDS
YOUR CHEST AS FAR AS YOU CAN

WITHOUT STRAINING YOUR SELF

 AND THEN LOWER IT GENTLY TO THE PILLOW

 AND PRESS YOUR HEAD ON THE PILLOW

FEELING THE STRETCH OF YOUR SPINE

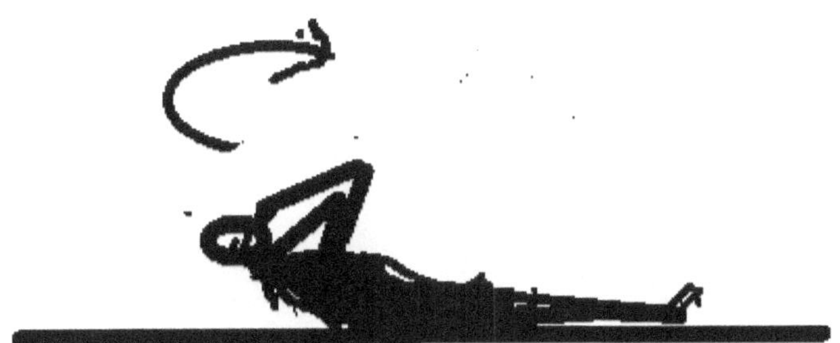

RAISE YOUR HEAD TO YOUR CHEST AS
MUCH AS YOU CAN WITHOUT STRAINING
YOURSELF,
AND THEN LET YOUR HEAD AND HANDS
GENTLY DOWN TO THE MATTRESS.

**REPEAT 5-10 TIMES AND KEEP
INCREASING THEM EVERY WEEK**

 **THIS EXERCISE STRETCHES
YOUR WHOLE SPINE**

4)KNEE TO CHEST

AND RAISE YOUR HEAD TOWARDS
YOUR KNEE

LYING FACE UP ,

  INTERLOCKED FINGERS UNDER
YOUR HEAD

AND LEGS EXTENDED FEET
TOGETHER ON THE MATTRESS

 A)BEND YOUR RIGHT KNEE

AND BRING IT TOWARDS YOUR
CHEST

 THEN RAISE YOUR HEAD
TOWARDS YOUR BEND KNEE

WITHOUT STRAINING YOURSELF

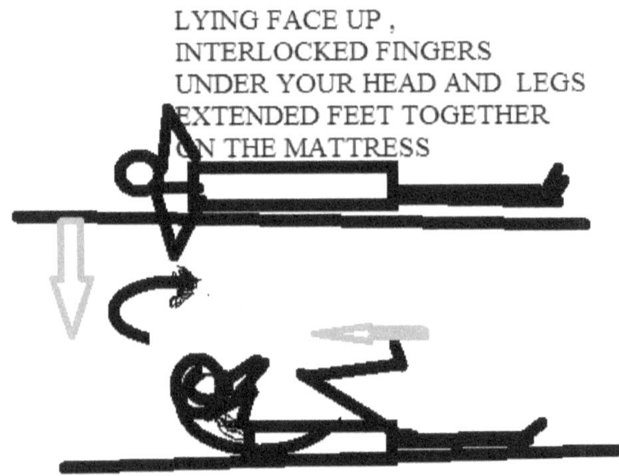

BEND YOUR RIGHT KNEE AND BRING IT TOWARDS YOUR
CHEST
THEN RAISE YOUR HEAD TOWARDS YOUR BEND KNEE
WITHOUT STRAINING YOURSELF

AND HOLD FOR THE COUNT OF TWO

LOWER YOUR HEAD GENTLY ON THE MATTRESS

AND EXTEND YOUR KNEE.

B)REPEAT THE SAME EXERCISE
WITH LEFT KNEE

THEN BEND YOUR LEFT KNEE

AND BRING IT TOWARDS YOUR
CHEST

THEN RAISE YOUR HEAD
TOWARDS YOUR KNEE

WITHOUT STRAINING YOURSELF,

HOLD THIS POSITION FOR THE
COUNT OF TWO

AND THEN LOWER YOUR HEAD
GENTLY TO THE MATTRESS

AND EXTEND YOUR KNEE.

5) BOTH   KNEES TO CHEST

**AND RAISING YOUR HEAD
TOWARDS KNEES**

LYING FACE UP ,

**INTERLOCKED FINGERS UNDER
YOUR HEAD**

BEND YOUR KNEES

**AND BRING THEM TO YOUR
CHEST**

AS CLOSE AS POSSIBLE

WITHOUT STRAINING G YOURSELF

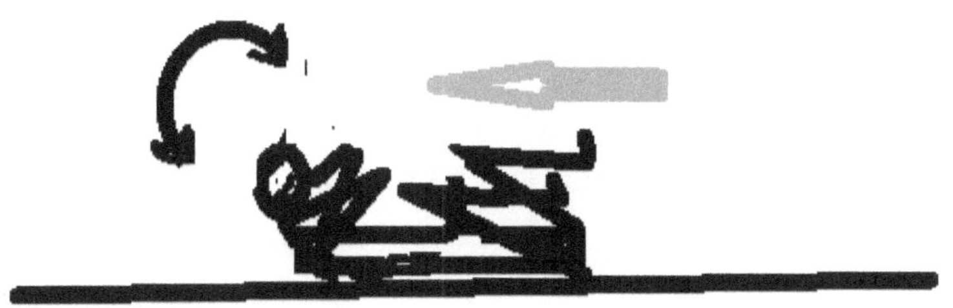

LYING FACE UP , INTERLOCKED FINGERS
UNDER YOUR HEAD
BEND YOUR KNEES AND BRING THEM TO
YOUR CHEST AS CLOSE AS POSSIBLE WITHOUT
STRAINING G YOURSELF
AND RAISE YOUR HEAD TOWARDS YOUR
KNEES

**AND RAISE YOUR HEAD TOWARDS
YOUR KNEES**

HOLD FOR THE COUNT OF TWO

**AND LOWER YOUR HEAD GENTLY
TO THE MATTRESS**

**AND YOUR BENT KNEES   TO THE
MATTRESS**

REPEAT THIS EXERCISE 5 TIMES

 **REST BY TAKING A DEEP
BREATH**

AND EXHALING SLOWLY

6) SPINAL ACTIVE FLEXION EXERCISE

BENT KNEE TO SIDE AND RAISING YOUR HEAD

LYING FACE UP,

YOUR INTERLOCKED FINGERS
UNDER YOUR HEAD

 AND YOUR KNEES BENT WITH
FEET FIRMLY FLAT ON THE
MATTRESS

   A)LET YOUR BENT RIGHT KNEE
SLIDE TO YOUR RIGHT SIDE
TOUCHING THE MATTRESS

THEN RAISE YOUR HEAD
TOWARDS YOUR CHEST

 WITHOUT STRAINING YOURSELF

 HOLD TO THE COUNT OF TWO

THEN LOWER YOUR HEAD GENTLY
TO THE MATTRESS

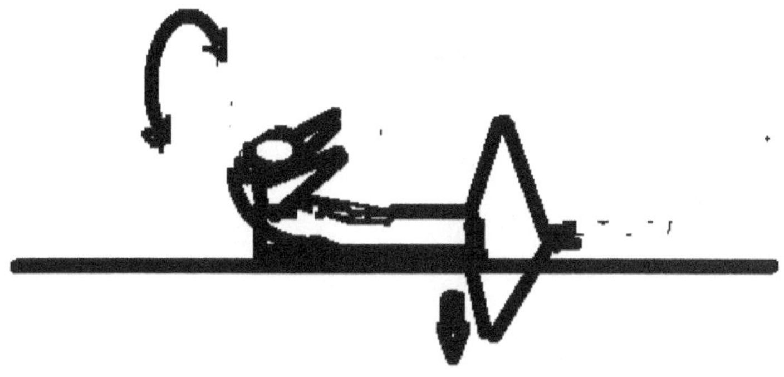

LET YOUR BENT RIGHT KNEE SLIDE TO YOUR
RIGHT SIDE TOUCHING THE MATTRESS
THEN RAISE YOUR HEAD TOWARDS YOUR CHEST
WITHOUT STRAINING YOURSELF
HOLD TO THE COUNT OF TWO
THEN LOWER YOUR HEAD GENTLY TO THE
MATTRESS AND YOUR RIGHT KNEE BACK UP TO
TOUCH THE LEFT KNEE

**AND YOUR RIGHT KNEE BACK UP
TO TOUCH THE LEFT KNEE**

**B) LET YOUR BENT LEFT KNEE
SLIDE TO YOUR LEFT SIDE TO
TOUCH THE MATTRESS**

**THEN RAISE YOUR HEAD
TOWARDS YOUR CHEST**

WITHOUT STRAINING YOUR SELF ,

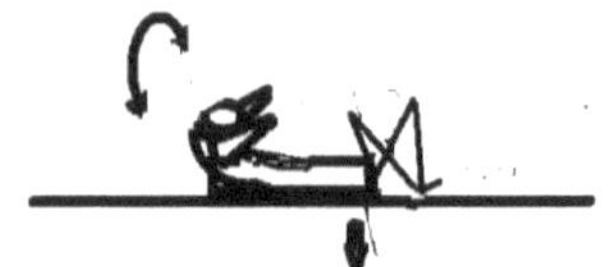

LET YOUR BENT RIGHT KNEE SLIDE TO YOUR
RIGHT SIDE TOUCHING THE MATTRESS
THEN RAISE YOUR HEAD TOWARDS YOUR CHEST
WITHOUT STRAINING YOURSELF
HOLD TO THE COUNT OF TWO
THEN LOWER YOUR HEAD GENTLY TO THE
MATTRESS AND YOUR RIGHT KNEE BACK UP TO
TOUCH THE LEFT KNEE

HOLD FOR THE COUNT OF TWO

THEN LOWER YOUR HEAD

**GENTLY TO THE MATTRESS
AND YOUR LEFT KNEE BACK UP
TO THE OTHER KNEE**

**REPEAT THIS EXERCISE 5 TIMES
EACH KNEE**

THIS EXERCISE IS VERY GOOD TO
MOBILIZE YOUR HIPS, PELVIC
JOINTS AND THE JOINTS OF
YOUR WHOLE SPINE

EVERY WEEK YOU INCREASE
THEM UNTIL YOU REACH 20-30

WITHOUT STRAINING YOURSELF.

7)RAISING YOUR LOW BACK
TOWARDS THE CEILING

LYING DOWN FACE UP WITH
YOUR KNEES BENT

AND YOUR HANDS   UNDER YOUR
HEAD

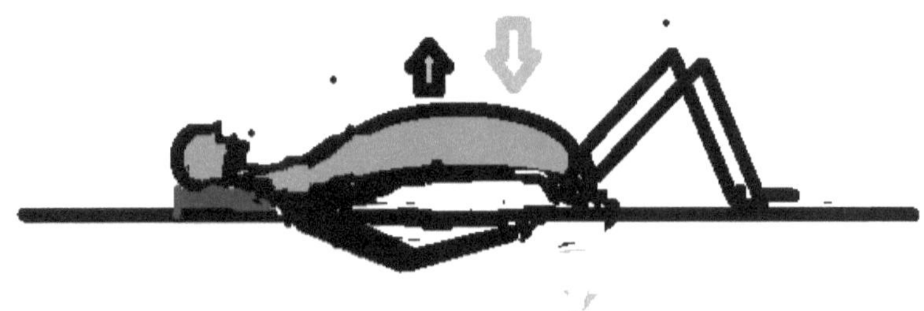

LYING DOWN FACE UP WITH YOUR KNEES BENT
AND YOUR HANDS ON THE SIDE BESIDES   YOUR LOW BACK
RAISE YOUR LOW BACK TOWARDS THE CEILING AND THEN
DOWN,
UP AND DOWN FOR 5-10 TIMES OR MORE WITHOUT YOUR
LOW BACK TOUCHING THE MATTRESS
AND THEN LOWER YOUR LOW BACK GENTLY TO THE
MATTRESS.

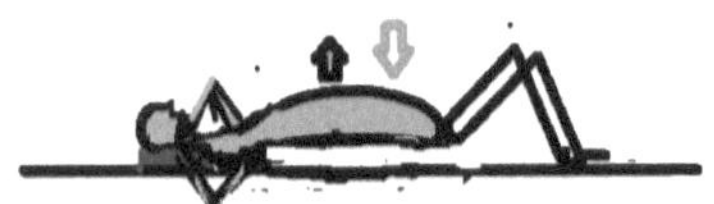

LYING DOWN FACE UP WITH YOUR KNEES BENT
AND YOUR ,INTELACED HANDS UNDER YOUR HEAD
RAISE YOUR LOW BACK TOWARDS THE CEILING AND THEN
DOWN,
UP AND DOWN FOR 5-10 TIMES OR MORE WITHOUT YOUR
LOW BACK TOUCHING THE MATTRESS
AND THEN LOWER YOUR LOW BACK GENTLY TO THE
MATTRESS.

RAISE YOUR LOW BACK TOWARDS
THE CEILING

 AND THEN DOWN, UP AND DOWN
FOR 5-10 TIMES

OR MORE WITHOUT YOUR LOW
BACK TOUCHING THE MATTRESS

 THEN LOWER YOUR LOW BACK
GENTLY TO THE MATTRESS.

REST BY TAKING   A BREATH OR
TWO

REPEAT THIS EXERCISE 10 TIMES

 AND EVERY WEEK YOU INCREASE
THEM UNTIL YOU REACH 20-30

WITHOUT STRAINING YOURSELF.

8) SPINAL ACTIVE FLEXION EXERCISES

KNEE TO CHEST   EXERCISE

LYING FACE UP WITH YOUR KNEES BENT
AND YOUR HANDS ON YOUR SIDE

A)DRAW YOUR RIGHT KNEE TO YOUR CHEST

GRAB IT WITH BOTH HANDS AND PRESS IT ON YOUR CHEST,

AND RAISE YOUR HEAD TOWARDS YOUR KNEE

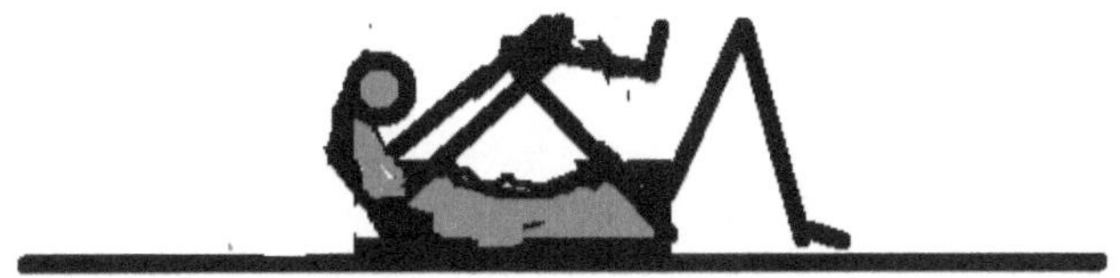

A)DRAW YOUR RIGHT KNEE TO YOUR CHEST
GRAB IT WITH BOTH HANDS AND PRESS IT ON YOUR CHEST,
AND RAISE YOUR HEAD TOWARDS YOUR KNEE

HOLD IT FOR THE COUNT OF TWO
 THEN RETURN IT TO ITS ORIGINAL BENT POSITION.

HOLD IT FOR THE COUNT OF TWO

THEN RETURN IT TO ITS ORIGINAL BENT POSITION

. B)   THEN FROM THE SAME POSITION

DRAW YOUR LEFT KNEE TO YOUR CHEST

GRASP IT WITH BOTH HANDS AND
PRESS IT ON YOUR CHEST

AND RAISE YOUR HEAD
TOWARDS YOUR KNEE

.HOLD IT FOR THE COUNT OF TWO

THEN RETURN IT TO ITS
ORIGINAL BENT POSITION.

REPEAT THIS EXERCISE 5-10
TIMES ON EACH KNEE THEN REST
FOR 2-3 MINUTES

9) KNEES TO CHEST EXERCISES

AND RAISE YOUR HEAD TOWARDS YOUR BENT KNEES

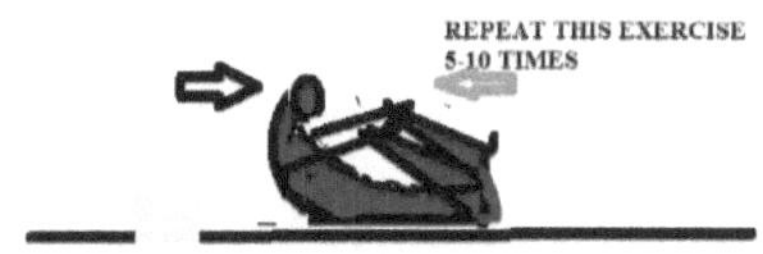

WITH YOUR KNEES BENT DRAW BOTH KNEES TO YOUR CHEST,
GRAB YOUR KNEES WITH BOTH HANDS DRAWING THE KNEES AS NEAR
TO THE CHEST AS POSSIBLE.
AND THEN RAISE YOUR HEAD TOWARDS YOUR KNEES

WITHOUT STRAINING YOURSELF

HOLD IT FOR THE COUNT OF TWO

THEN LOWER YOUR HEAD GENTLY TO THE MATTRESS
AND YOUR FEET TO THE MATTRESS

FROM THE SAME POSITION

LYING FACE UP

WITH YOUR KNEES BENT

DRAW BOTH KNEES TO YOUR CHEST,

GRAB YOUR KNEES WITH BOTH HANDS

DRAWING THE KNEES AS NEAR TO THE CHEST AS POSSIBLE.

AND THEN RAISE YOUR HEAD TOWARDS YOUR KNEES

WITHOUT STRAINING YOURSELF

HOLD IT FOR THE COUNT OF TWO

THEN LOWER YOUR HEAD GENTLY TO THE MATTRESS

AND YOUR FEET TO THE MATTRESS

DO THIS EXERCISE 5-10 TIMES

WITHOUT STRAINING YOURSELF

10)KNEES TO CHEST ROCKING EXERCISE

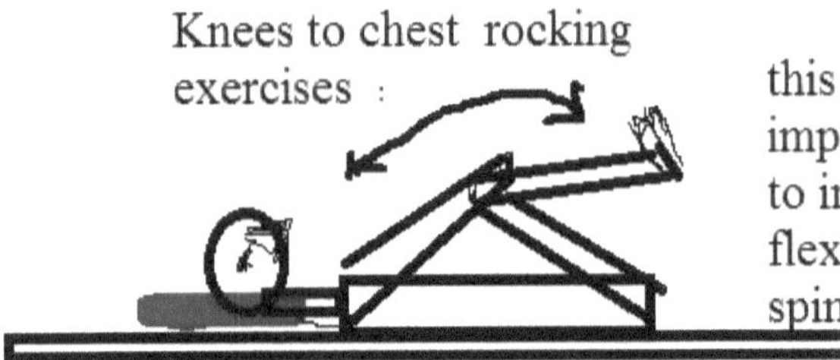

grab your right knee with your right
hand and your left knee with your left
hand and bring your knees to your
chest and with a rocking motion rock
your pelvis back and forth

LYING FACE UP WITH YOUR KNEES BENT

AND YOUR HANDS ON YOUR SIDE

BRING YOUR BENT KNEES TOWARDS YOUR CHEST

GRASP YOUR RIGHT KNEE WITH YOUR RIGHT HAND

AND YOUR LEFT KNEE WITH YOUR LEFT HAND

AND PRESS THEM ON YOUR CHEST,

WHILE HOLDING YOUR KNEES ABOUT 6 INCHES APART WITH YOUR HANDS

WITH A ROCKING MOVE

ROCK YOUR PELVIS BACK AND FORTH

BY BRING YOUR KNEES TO YOUR CHEST

AND BACK WITHOUT YOUR FEET TOUCHING THE MATTRESS

REPEAT THIS EXERCISE 10-20 TIMES

WITHOUT STRAINING YOUR SELF

AND INCREASE EVERY WEEK BY
5 MORE TIMES

UNTIL YOU CAN EASILY DO 100.

REST FOR A FEW SECONDS
OR MORE DEPENDING HOW YOU
FEEL

BY TAKING DEEP BREATHS

AND EXHALING SLOWLY.

REMEMBER NOT TO OVERDO IT
WITH THE EXERCISES.

START SLOWLY WITH A FEW AND
INCREASING THEM

AS YOU GET STRONGER

THIS IS A VERY IMPORTANT
EXERCISE, AND THIS IS THE
MAXIMUM BEND FORWARD THAT
MIMICS THE ADAMS TEST

STRETCHING THE SPINE TO ITS
MAXIMUM WITHOUT GRAVITY.

 THIS EXERCISE MOBILIZES ALL
JOINTS OF THE SPINE, HIP AND
PELVIS JOINTS AND CHEST AND
SHOULDER JOINTS

11) SPINAL STRETCH MIMICKING

THE BICYCLES PEDALING MOVES

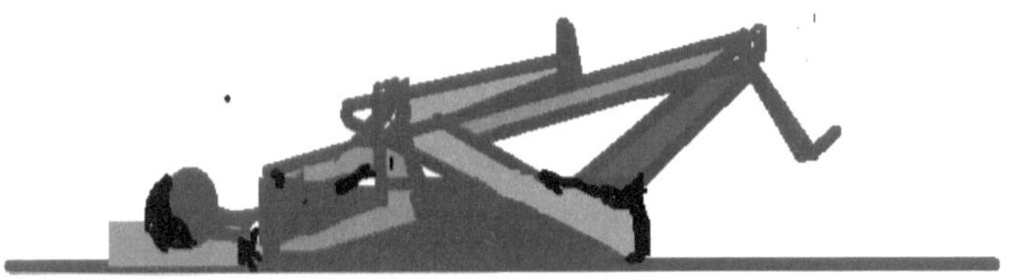

WHILE HOLDING YOUR KNEES ABOUT 6 INCHES APART WITH YOUR HANDS
BRING YOUR LEFT KNEE UP TOWARDS YOUR CHEST
AND SIMULTANEOUSLY PUSH YOUR RIGHT KNEE DOWN TOWARDS THE
MATTRESS WITHOUT TOUCHING THE MATTRESS
WHILE YOU STILL HOLD YOUR KNEES
AND KEEP MOVING ONE KNEE UP AND THE OTHER DOWN MIMICKING THE
PEDALING OF A BICYCLE

**LYING FACE UP WITH YOUR
KNEES BENT**

AND YOUR HANDS BY YOUR SIDE

**BRING YOUR BENT KNEES
TOWARDS YOUR CHEST**

**GRASP YOUR RIGHT KNEE WITH
YOUR RIGHT HAND**

AND YOUR LEFT KNEE WITH
YOUR LEFT HAND

AND   WHILE HOLDING YOUR
KNEES ABOUT 6 INCHES APART

WITH YOUR HANDS

BRING YOUR LEFT KNEE UP
TOWARDS YOUR CHEST

AND SIMULTANEOUSLY PUSH
YOUR RIGHT KNEE

DOWN TOWARDS THE MATTRESS
WITHOUT TOUCHING THE
MATTRESS

WHILE YOU STILL HOLD YOUR
KNEES

AND KEEP MOVING ONE KNEE UP

AND THE OTHER DOWN

MIMICKING THE PEDALING OF A BICYCLE

KEEP DOING IT FOR THE COUNT OF FIFTY ,

WHICH IS ABOUT A MINUTE,

BUT DO NOT EXERT YOURSELF.

12) SPINAL STRETCH

WHILE LYING DOWN FACE UP.

**EXTEND YOUR HANDS ABOVE
YOUR HEAD**

**TRYING TO REACH AS FAR AS YOU
CAN**

**AND SIMULTANEOUSLY   WITH
YOUR FEET   TOGETHER
TOUCHING THE MATTRESS**

**STRETCH THEM DOWN AS FAR AS
YOU CAN**

EXTEND YOUR HANDS ABOVE YOUR HEAD TRYING
TO REACH AS FAR AS YOU CAN
AND SIMULTANEOUSLY
 WITH YOUR FEET   TOGETHER TOUCHING THE
MATTRESS STRETCH THEM DOWN AS FAR AS
YOU CAN

THIS IS A SPINAL STRETCH EXERCISE
FEEL THE SPINAL STRETCH

TAKE A DEEP BREATH

EXPANDING YOUR CHEST AS
MUCH AS POSSIBLE

THIS IS A SPINAL STRETCH
EXERCISE

FEEL THE SPINAL STRETCH

EXHALE SLOWLY,

REPEAT 5 TIME

N.B. If there are no
contraindications you can ALSO
do the Adams forward flexion
exercise during the day.

13)ADAMS BEND FORWARDS TEST EXERCISE

START WITH THE STANDING POSITION,

FEET AND KNEES TOGETHER,

BEND FORWARD TRYING TO REACH YOUR TOES WITH THE FINGERS OF YOUR HANDS

ADAMS BEND FORWARDS TEST EXERCISE

START WITH THE STANDING POSITION, FEET AND KNEES TOGETHER, BEND FORWARD TRYING TO REACH YOUR TOES WITH THE FINGERS OF YOUR HANDS

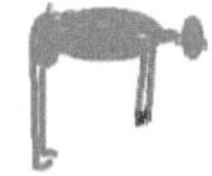

THIS EXERCISE STRETCHES YOUR WHOLE SPINE AND THE SPINE STRAIGHTENS IN FUNCTIONAL SCOLIOSIS. AND TRIES TO STRAIGHTEN IN STRUCTURAL SCOLIOSIS

THIS EXERCISE STRETCHES YOUR WHOLE SPINE

  AND THE SPINE STRAIGHTENS IN FUNCTIONAL SCOLIOSIS.

  AND TRIES TO STRAIGHTEN IN STRUCTURAL SCOLIOSIS.

14) MODIFIED ADAMS FORWARD BEND TEST EXERCISE

  START WITH THE STANDING POSITION

  BUT YOUR FEET ARE PLACED 12-18 INCHES APART

BEND FORWARDS

**AND TOUCH YOUR LEFT FOOT
WITH YOUR RIGHT HAND FINGERS**

**WHILE YOUR LEFT HAND IS AT
THE BACK OF YOUR LOW BACK**

START WITH THE STANDING POSITION BUT
YOUR FEET ARE PLACED 12-18 INCHES APART
BEND FORWARDS AND TOUCH YOUR LEFT
FOOT WITH YOUR RIGHT HAND FINGERS
WHILE YOUR LEFT HAND RESTS ON THE BACK
OF YOUR LOW BACK

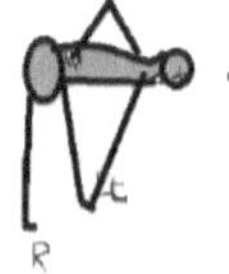

**YOU COME UP TO STRAIGHT
POSITION**

**AND THEN BEND FORWARDS AND
TOUCH YOUR RIGHT FOOT**

WITH YOUR LEFT HAND FINGERS

NB. IF YOU HAVE A NOTICEABLE
RIB HUMP

ON YOUR RIGHT SIDE,

THEN DO TWICE AS MANY BENDS

 WITH YOUR RIGHT HAND TO
YOUR LEFT FOOT

AND VICE VERSA.

THIS IS DONE BECAUSE WHEN
YOU BRING YOUR RIGHT HAND (
THE SIDE OF YOUR HUMP) TO
YOUR LEFT FOOT THE BENDING
STRETCH DRAWS FORWARD YOUR
HUMP AND CORRECTS YOUR RIB
CAGE

AND WITH TIME IT SHOULD BRING
IT BACK TO NORMAL ,THAT'S WHY

YOU DO THE BENDS TWICE AS
MUCH ON THE SIDE OF HUMP.

DO THESE EXERCISES   3 TIMES A
DAY

 UNLESS YOU ARE SICK OR HAVE
FEVER IN WHICH CASE YOU DO
NOT DO ANY EXERCISES

THESE ARE THE MAIN EXERCISES
 BASED ON THE ADAMS BEND
FORWARD TEST, THAT WILL HELP
YOUR SCOLIOSIS

BUT YOU HAVE TO DO THEM
EVERY DAY RELIGIOUSLY

3 TIMES A DAY, MORNING WHEN
YOU WAKE UP AND TWICE IN THE
AFTERNOON

AS WITH ANY OTHER EXERCISES ,
 YOU EXERCISE ON AN EMPTY
STOMACH.

AND TAKE IT EASY AT THE
BEGINNING
 UNTIL YOUR BODY GETS
STRONGER, FLEXIBLE AND YOU
HAVE MORE ENDURANCE

 OTHER EXERCISES THAT WILL
HELP YOU STRAIGHTEN OUT
YOUR SPINE ARE

THE MONKEY BAR WHICH I
HIGHLY RECOMMEND

 YOU USE ANY TIME YOU HAVE
THE CHANCE

.MAYBE EVERYDAY

15) USE A MONKEY BAR TO
EXERCISE.

 WHICH IS VERY GOOD FOR
STRETCHING YOUR SPINE

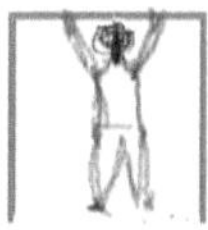

EXERCISING
ON THE
MONKEY BAR

   GRAB THE MONKEY BAR WITH
BOTH HANDS

 AND LET YOUR BODY SWING BACK
AND FORTH A FEW TIMES,

AND YOU CAN DO SOME CHIN UPS IF YOU WANT

.REPEAT IT OFTEN WITHOUT STRAINING YOURSELF.

THIS EXERCISE STRETCHES YOUR SPINE NATURALLY WITH YOUR OWN BODY. WEIGHT...

BESIDES MONKEYS DO IT ALL THE TIME

AND THEY NEVER GET SCOLIOSIS.

16) SWIMMING IS AN EXCELLENT EXERCISE FOR SCOLIOSIS.

TRY TO SWIM 1-2 TIMES A WEEK
IF YOU CAN.

I HIGHLY RECOMMEND IT.

SWIMMING EXERCISES ALL THE
MUSCLES OF THE BODY

AND I HIGHLY RECOMMEND IT.

BESIDES FISHES THAT SWIM ALL
THE TIME,

DO NOT GET SCOLIOSIS .

17)WALKING IS AN EXCELLENT
EXERCISE

MAKE IT A HABIT TO WALK DAILY
WITHOUT SLOUCHING.

BE PROUD OF YOUR BODY AND
YOUR POSTURE!

 BUT NOT FOR PEOPLE WITH TRAUMA, PATHOLOGY OR HAD SURGERY AND RODS.
 IT IS VERY GOOD FOR PEOPLE WITH FUNCTIONAL SCOLIOSIS BUT IT WILL HELP ONLY IF PEOPLE WITH SCOLIOSIS CHANGE THEIR DAILY BAD POSTURAL HABITS AVOID BAD SITTING HABITS AND THEY SHOULD SIT STRAIGHT ON A CHAIR AT HOME AT SCHOOL, AND AVOID SLOUCHING, WHEN THEY WATCH TV OR PLAY VIDEO GAMES AND NEVER CARY HEAVY OBJECTS ON ONE SIDE OF THEIR BODY, SUCH AS HEAVY BACK PACKS ,OR BABIES............

DISCLAIMER:

THIS IS FOR INFORMATION ONLY AND
 NOT TO GIVE ANY MEDICAL ADVICE .
YOU SHOULD NOT HAVE ANY PAIN WHILE DOING THE EXERCISES.
 IF YOU HAVE ANY PAIN SEE YOUR DOCTOR

.....REMEMBER, PEOPLE THAT EXERCISE DAILY HAVE GOOD POSTURE, GOOD HEALTH .A STRONG HEALTHY AND FLEXIBLE SPINE

 AND NEVER GET SCOLIOSIS.....

 I NEVER SAW ANY   BODY BUILDER
OR ANY OTHER ATHLETE THAT EXERCISES DAILY   WITH SCOLIOSIS.

THE SOLUTION TO THIS PREVENTABLE CONDITION CALLED SCOLIOSIS IS SIMPLY ,EXERCISE DAILY   AND NOT ANY MAGIC PILL INVENTED IN A LABORATORY...

I RECENTLY WATCHED A VIDEO ON YOU TUBE , MADE IN 2018 ,BY ARNOLD SCHWARZENEGGER AND SYLVESTER STALLONE EXERCISING, AND I THINK THEY ARE IN THEIR 70S, AND ARNOLD SAID " YOU HAVE TO EXERCISE DAILY".

 LOOK AT THE SHAPE THEY ARE IN THEIR 70S?

 DO YOU THINK THAT THOSE GUYS AND OTHERS THAT EXERCISE DAILY, COULD GET A SCOLIOSIS IN THEIR SPINE?

I DO NOT THINK SO.

Every day millions of people are doing some of the exercises i described above, or similar exercises, in the gyms , the military training their soldiers, at the beaches swimming, at schools and at home and they have strong healthy and flexible spines The only thing they have not realized is that these exercises helped them to avoid abnormal curves in their spines, scoliosis, kyphosis and lordosis.If the people that got scoliosis or any other abnormal curve, they were doing the right exercises , like the S.A.FE. I describe above they would also have a strong , healthy , flexible spine without any abnormal curves.
  EVEN after they got the abnormal curves, if they start exercising, their spine will get stronger , more flexible and with time they might reverse that abnormal curve, or at least stop the progression of that abnormal curve, if it is not that severe that requires surgery.

CHAPTER TEN

SUMMARY OF THE DAILY ROUTINE   HOME EXERCISES " S.A.F.E". SPINAL FLEXION EXERCISES

IN SUMMARY THIS IS THE DAILY ROUTINE FOR THE S.A.F.E. EXERCISES.

START SLOWLY AND EASY AND AS YOU GET STRONGER AND

MORE FLEXIBLE INCREASE THE TIMES YOU DO THESE EXERCISES.

 NEVER OVER DO IT AND NEVER STRAIN YOURSELF. BUILD UP YOUR ENDURANCE OVER TIME!

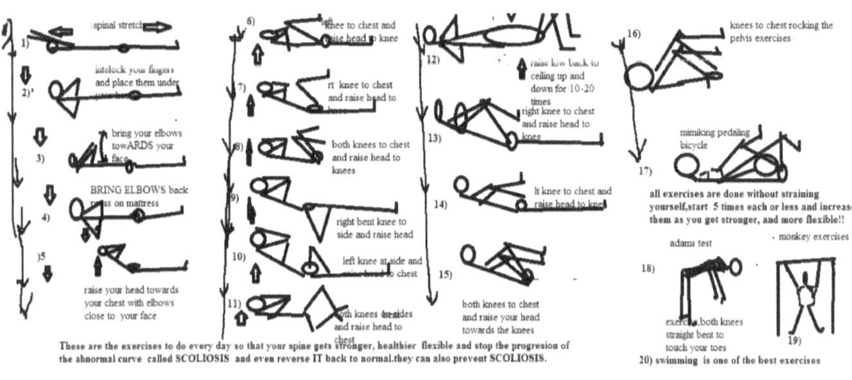

Regular exercise is important for children with scoliosis. It can help improve muscle strength and may help reduce the scoliosis and pain.

Children with scoliosis can usually do most types of exercise safely. They only need to avoid certain activities   such as lifting heavy objects or backpacks, and sit straight on the chair at home and school and avoid bad sitting or slouching when they watch TV or play video games. Poor posture and slouching should be avoided and never carry on the side of their body or shoulder.

 Specific back exercises .such as the ones. I designed the S.A.F.E. exercises to help improve scoliosis by strengthening the back muscles and the flexibility of the spine.

Many children won't need any other treatment, provided that they exercise every day and avoid bad postural habits .Only a small number will end up having surgery if their scoliosis was advanced before starting the exercises.

 Children and young people should also reduce the time they spend sitting for extended periods of time,

watching TV, playing computer
games and other   prolong sitting
activities.

GOOD LUCK TO ALL.

CHAPTER ELEVEN

EXPECTED RESULTS

The S.A.F.E . exercises are designed to give flexibility and strength to the spine as long as you do them daily.

To have good results you have to change your old habits of bad posture at home, at school and everywhere else.

 If you do the exercises and keep doing what you have been doing that started the scoliosis, do not expect much, because you did not remove the CAUSE that started the scoliosis.

You might see some improvement but not as much as   when you removed the cause, the bad posture habits. .

if you do the exercises daily three times a day and you removed the cause of the scoliosis, and if you are a girl you should stop lifting and carrying babies around , with these exercises along with some swimming exercises and   monkey bar stretching exercises you should get good results in 2-3 months .

Even when you see some improvement you should keep doing the exercises daily for ever if you want to have a strong ,healthy, flexible spine, along with all the other benefits that come with a healthy spine. It will be taking you about 15 minutes times 3 a total of 45 minutes a day and the health benefits   are good.

 Of course you will be doing these exercises on an empty stomach and you should not exercise when you are sick with fever , infections or have pain.

 I am not a believer of "NO PAIN NO GAIN."

When there is pain it is a warning from your body to stop and you should always listen to your body.

CHAPTER TWELVE

RESEARCH:

Research is needed to identify the
real multiple causes of the so called
IDIOPATHIC SCOLIOSIS which is
not idiopathic at all , they just did
not recognize the cause.

To call it IDIOPATHIC and do
nothing about it while we watch it
to get worse   ruining the lives of
millions of youngsters I think it is
not a good   thing to do.

Or just believe in wild THEORIES
that scoliosis is caused by the
bones growing faster than the
nerve trunks and the nerve trunks
are pulling the bones into a
scoliotic curve is absurd.

IF that was the case every time the
surgeons fuse the spine and put
rods to correct the scoliosis the
nerve trunks would break leaving
the patient with severe
catastrophic neurological problems

including paralysis, something
which thankfully is not happening
now.

Yes, I watched this video on YOU
TUBE, a medical doctor holding a
spine and pulling some strings to
cause a scoliosis, claiming that was
the real cause of IDIOPATHIC
scoliosis according to the theory of
some dr. Roth , that the bones are
growing faster than the nerve
trunks causing the spine into
scoliosis.

Fortunately it is just a theory and I
hope that not many doctors believe
in that absurd theory, otherwise
they will throw their hands up in
the air and say there is nothing we
can do about scoliosis and stop the
search to reverse the abnormal
curve.

 WITH ALL THE ADVANCES IN
TECHNOLOGY WE CAN EASILY
IDENTIFY, AT LEAST WITH
STATISTICS, WHAT'S CAUSING
WHAT.

 With the help of statistics we can
know how many women had babies

the natural way and what percentage of those babies develop infantile scoliosis. How many women had babies with the use of instrumentation and how many of those babies develop scoliosis, wry neck or had other health problems such as cerebral palsy etc.

How many women had their babies with cesarean section and how many of those babies develop scoliosis or other health problems? By analyzing those statistics we can see which method of delivering the babies is the most safe and causes less health problems to the mother and the baby, and if a woman has a difficult delivery instead of waiting and using instruments with the possibility to cause injuries to the new baby, let her have a cesarean section delivery instead.

How many kids are diagnoses with infantile scoliosis after a normal birth and under what conditions.

Give the mothers a questionnaire
to fill out and see what is the
common cause that causes the
infantile scoliosis. Falls, injuries ,
or just bad positioning of the baby?
when you recognize the common
cause , name the scoliosis with that
cause.
Such as POSITIONAL INFANTILE
SCOLIOSIS when it is caused by
bad positioning of the baby, or,
 TRAUMATIC INFANTILE
SCOLIOSIS when there is an injury
or fall that caused the scoliosis,
 AND treat each condition
accordingly.

 With juvenile idiopathic scoliosis
again try to find the cause and
name the scoliosis accordingly.
when we have a cause and a name
it is easier to treat. Give the kids
and their parents a questionnaire
about their lifestyle and habits and
see if there are common elements ,
in lifestyle or habits that cause the
scoliosis and name it accordingly.
BAD POSTURAL POSITIONS
JUVENILE SCOLIOSIS, simply
POSTURAL JUVENILE SCOLIOSIS
if it is due to daily bad postural
positions, like slouching on the

sofa watching television , studying,
playing video games etc.

 OR KIDS PLAYING WITH
BABIES NAME IT 'BABYSITTING
JUVENILE SCOLIOSIS ', if the kids
baby-sit play with their siblings
,nephews or other babies for long
periods of time.

 Statistics can help identify the
cause and when the cause is known
it is not IDIOPATHIC ANYMORE,
and by just eliminating the cause of
the new named scoliosis and give
them the right spinal stretching
exercises the scoliosis will improve
, even eliminated????.

Any research done it has to involve
the youngsters that have the
scoliosis to find the cause and
eliminate whatever the cause is.

Any research done in the laboratory
searching for genes or other causes
without the involvement of those
who already have the condition will
not have any meaningful use in

the treatment and correction of
the abnormal curve. Looking at
DNA markers for scoliosis and start
performing surgeries on healthy
youngsters that have the so called
DNA markers but no scoliosis yet,
just with the laboratory theory
that you will prevent future
scoliosis it is absurd .
 If , however use the DNA markers
to encourage the youngsters to
exercise and prevent them from
developing scoliosis, that would be
acceptable.

   Based on the observations of
William Adams that he observed
,that a scoliotic spine tries to
straighten out when bending
forward(flexion of the spine) " the
Adams forward bend test ," I
devised specific spinal exercises
for repeat flexion of the spine
without the gravity, simply lying
face up while doing the exercises,.

 I hope that with these exercises
which I call them   SPINAL ACTIVE
FLEXION EXERCISES, S.A.F.E. will
help a lot of people that have

scoliosis and other curvatures,
kyphosis and lordosis and help a lot
of other youngsters to prevent
them from developing scoliosis.

 It is my hope that the government
or other organization that have
the funds and the human resources
will contact   a research   to prove
how effective my designed
exercises   are in treating and
preventing the abnormal curvatures
of the spine, scoliosis, kyphosis
and lordosis.

 With the technological means we
have these days the research can be
done over the internet over a
period of six months to a year.
There are millions of youngsters
diagnosed with scoliosis of various
degrees every year.

Take 10,000 youngsters   that are
diagnosed with scoliosis and
instead of advising them "to wait
and see "in six months or a year ,
 divide them into   5
groups

1)The first group of 2000 youngsters, just advise them to wait and see what happen in a year ,nothing else .

 THIS IS THE STANDARD ADVISE THEY GIVE THE YOUNGSTERS NOW!

 2)the second group of 2000 youngsters advised them to just change their postural positional lifestyle.. and start to sit properly while at school and home, avoid slouching positions while watching television for the next six months to a year.

3)the third group of 2000 youngsters advise them to avoid their bad positions lifestyle and start doing the S.A.F.E. exercises I designed based on the Adams forward bend test of the spine, the repeated flexion of the spine without gravity., lying face up while they do the exercises.

 4)the fourth group of 2000 youngsters advised them to avoid their bad positioning habits, start doing the exercises I designed S.A.F.E. and add   swimming and monkey bar stretching exercises

 5)the fifth group of 2000 youngsters after they are diagnosed with scoliosis just advise them to do only the S.A.F.E. exercises daily for six months to a year.

 At the end of six months OR one year, check the x-rays of the youngsters and see which group of youngsters have any improvement in their abnormal scoliosis curve and which group   stay the same and which group   got worse .

THE RESULTS WILL SPEAK FOR THEMSELVES.

My prediction is:

 that group one   their scoliosis will
get worse, ;they did nothing to
help their scoliosis, and they will be
doing exactly what they have bee
doing to cause the scoliosis in the
first place. So   unless something
dramatic changed in their daily
lifestyle habits they will have a
worse condition in their spinal
curvature.

 Group 2   their scoliosis might be
the same or have some
improvement. At least they
changed their bad postural habits,
provided they did.

Group 3 their scoliosis should show
a lot of improvement and even
reverse somewhat. They changed
their bad postural habits plus they
were doing the S.A.F.E.
EXERCISES which are very good
in strengthening their spinal
muscles   and increase their spinal
flexibility.

Group 4 of youngsters their
scoliosis should improve a lot and
even reverse to almost normal
depending on how bad it was when
they started and how often they
do the exercises.

This is the ideal situation for the
prevention and treatment of
scoliosis.

Group 5 of youngsters should have
some improvement but not as much
as much as group 4 which , they
stopped the bad habits and they
were doing swimming and monkey
bar exercises.

The S.A.F.E exercises are very
good for prevention and treatment
of scoliosis but with the
complementary exercises of the
monkey bar exercises and
swimming you get better results in
a shorter period of time.

Considering the huge amounts of money that every year the governments and other organizations spend, trying to find a cure for scoliosis ,this research will be easy and cheap to carry out as it can be done over the internet no matter where the youngsters are.

 Consider also the huge amounts of money that will be saved by the governments and the patients, if the cure for scoliosis, or just to stop the progression of the spinal abnormal curve is just to do home the S.A.F.E. exercises ,THE MONKEY BAR   AND SWIMMING and nothing else,

 NO UNCOMFORTABLE BRACES OR RISKY SURGERY OR OTHER EXPENSIVE AND TIME CONSUMING THERAPIES.

Wouldn't that be wonderful for the youngsters and all the people that suffer from scoliosis?

THE FUTURE WILL PROVE IF
THE "ADAMS FORWARD BEND"
TEST AND THE S.A.F.E.
EXERCISES I DESIGNED BASED ON
THAT OBSERVATION IS THE
MAGIC SOLUTION WE HAVE BEEN
LOOKING FOR SO LONG TO HELP
THE PEOPLE WITH SCOLIOSIS ,

GIVE THEM A TRY

AND   DON'T RUSH TO dismiss
them.

YOU MIGHT BE SURPRISED WITH
THE RESULTS!

MILLIONS OF ATHLETES AND
OTHER PEOPLE EXERCISING
DAILY DOING SOME OF MY
EXERCISES OR SIMILAR
EXERCISES IN THEIR DAILY
ROUTINE ALONG WITH SWIMMING
THE MONKEY BAR OR BODY

BUILDING EXERCISES, HAVE
STRONG, HEALTHY AND FLEXIBLE
SPINES WITHOUT ANY ABNORMAL
SPINAL CURVES!

I SIMPLY LIKE TO DRAW THE
ATTENTION TO ANYONE THAT
HAS SCOLIOSIS OR DIAGNOSES
AND TREATS PEOPLE WITH
SCOLIOSIS THAT EXERCISES IS A
GOOD OPTION   TO PREVENT AND
TREAT SCOLIOSIS.

   IT IS   100% BETTER OPTION
THAN THE ONE THAT THEY GIVE
TO PEOPLE NOW WHEN THEY
FIRST ARE DIAGNOSED WITH
SCOLIOSIS, THE SO CALLED "
WAIT AND SEE WHAT HAPPENS IN
SIX MONTHS OR A YEAR"

   I KNOW THAT MY DESIGNED
EXERCISES   S.A.F.E. WILL MAKE
ANY SPINE   STRONGER ,
FLEXIBLE AND STOP THE
PROGRESSION OF SCOLIOSIS
PROVIDED THAT PEOPLE WILL DO
THEM EVERY DAY............

BUT WHAT IF THE S.A.F.E.
EXERCISES ALSO REVERSE
COMPLETELY SOME FORMS OF
SCOLIOSIS SUCH AS THE
FUNCTIONAL SCOLIOSIS AND HELP
SOMEWHAT ALL TYPES OF
SCOLIOSIS, KYPHOSIS AND
LORDOSIS AND MAKE THE LIVES
OF PEOPLE BETTER?

DON'T YOU THINK THAT IT IS
WORTH INVESTIGATING THAT
POSSIBILITY WITH RESEARCH?

The solution to this preventable
condition known as SCOLIOSIS, is
prevention with good postural
habits at home at school, at work
and daily exercising to have a
strong, flexible and healthy spine.

The SPARTANS of ancient Greece
proved that   with their well
trained soldiers. the BODY
BUILDERS and the trained
athletes that exercise everyday
PROVE IT IN OUR TIMES.

CHAPTER THIRTEEN

PREVENTION OF SCOLIOSIS

There is a saying that "an once of prevention is worth a ton of therapy."

The best way to prevent scoliosis is exercise , the right exercises and avoid what causes scoliosis which can start as early as soon as a child is born.

As soon as a child is born the doctors and nurses that look after the mother and the child they should give the right instructions to the mother and those that are going to care for the baby how to look after the baby. instructions how to hold the baby to avoid the beginning of scoliosis to the mother and baby. NOT TO HOLD THE BABY ON ONE SIDE OF HER BODY, CAUSING SCOLIOSIS TO HER AND HER BABY.

NEVER TO PUT THE BABY FACE DOWN TO SLEEP,

**HAVE THE BABY SLEEP ON HIS
BACK OR HIS SIDE**

**BUT NEVER ALWAYS ONE SIDE, TO
AVOID THE MALFORMATION OF
THE BABY'S FACE OR SKULL.**

**BECAUSE THE BONES OF HIS
SKULL ARE STILL SOFT**

**NEVER TO LET OTHER KIDS TO
HOLD THE BABY ,**

**THEY MIGHT DROP THE BABY
CAUSING INJURIES ETC AND
MIGHT CAUSE STRAINS TO THE
OTHER KIDS SPINE STARTING A
SCOLIOSIS TO THE KIDS.**

**The parents should take good care
of their babies and if they notice an
abnormality to their face , spine,
hips or legs should take them to
their doctor for examination and
advice.**

The feet are the foundation of the whole body
and any abnormalities in the feet will affect the

whole body and possible cause a scoliosis to
develop.
It is very important to take good care of the
legs and feet of the babies to prevent future
problems in the skeletal system including the
pelvis and the spine.
When the babies use pampers diapers   , before
their toilet training, it is very important to
change the size of the pampers diapers as the
baby grows.
if the pampers diapers are too small they will
affect the circulation to the babies legs and
might cause some problems even an abnormal
short leg!
The mother might notice that her child is
limping while walking or that one leg is more
fad than the other due to the constriction of
the tight   diapers pampers.

IF THE BABIES develop an in-toeing or out-
toeing in their feet and walk with their toes
pointing inwards, .pigeon-toed walking
Or outwards the so called out-toe
walking or **duck-footed**
 The solution might just be to wear their shoes
opposite, in other words the left shoe to the
right foot and the right shoe to the left shoe
especially at night when they sleep and a few
hours when they walk for a while until there is
an improvement to their walking.
It is also a good idea to exercise the baby with

gentle the knees to chest exercises and take the
right foot and bring it gently to the left
shoulder and the left foot to the right shoulder.
These exercises will correct any tibia or
femoral twisting that might exist at the femoral
head causing the feet to turn outwards or
inwards.

**The parents should teach their
kids by example how to sit
properly at the dinner table, while
they study, or watching television,
or playing video games. They
should encourage the kids from
young age to exercise more by
taking them walking in the park,
bicycling, swimming and other
activities.**

**I WAS SURPRISED BUT VERY
PLEASED TO SEE RECENTLY ON
TELEVISION A PEDIATRICIAN
GIVING A YOUNG MOTHER A
PRESCRIPTION FOR HER CHILD '
TO DO MORE EXERCISES''.**

Kids should learn from an early age that exercises are good and necessary for good health!

If their kids are diagnosed with scoliosis and they were told to wait and see how it will develop they should encourage them to do the exercises above, enroll them in swimming classes 1-2 times a week and   use of a monkey bar to stretch their spine.

If they wait and see the possibility of the abnormal spine will get worse and might need braces and even surgery?

The teachers by example should encourage the kids to sit properly while they sit in the classroom.

The schools should have playgrounds with monkey bars and encourage the kids to use them.

The schools should   have   at least one session of spinal exercises like the ones I described above every day for 15-20 minutes.

I put a lot of emphasis on the school system, because their students spend a lot of time in schools sitting all day in classes and if they   sit in slouching positions and do no exercises there is a possibility that they will get an abnormal postural scoliosis.

Schools should have a scoliosis screening of their students at the beginning and end of each year .

The screening can be done by the school nurse or the gym teacher. A simple plumb line and   the Adams's bending forward test will be enough to do the screening and if a scoliosis is detected, or suspected, to refer the student to their doctor.   Any students that are diagnosed with scoliosis should do the S.A.F.E. exercises I designed above or similar exercises with swimming and the monkey bar stretching exercises.

It is my understanding, from reading the articles in the dangerous curve,:" A Dangerous Curve: The Role of History in America's ,"other industrialized nations (e.g., Canada, Great Britain, and Australia) that have overturned the long tradition of mandatory spinal screening of its school-aged citizens.4   ''

 that Australia, Canada , England and. many states in   the United States and other nations discontinued the scoliosis screening in schools because they had complaints about the screening process and   that they did not have any benefit in continuing the scoliosis screening.

 In the dangerous curve ,there was a picture of a woman   with a pen and a clipboard sitting in front of an almost nude girl doing the Adams test and I was wondering what the hell that woman was doing and if she had any training to do the Adams test? That woman was violating the privacy of that girl by having her exposed her underdeveloped chest and if that's how they were conducting the Adams test to all the young girls, I think there were many complaints from the young girls and their parents and rightly so.

The Adams test is done standing behind the child doing the test to observe the spine and not sitting in frond of the child, and in the case of the girls,   have them wear a gown or just their shirt backwards to expose only their spine, that's what you are testing.

 As for the tests effectiveness and not getting the desirable results to prevent or treat scoliosis I have to agree that the test is only for identify the scoliosis and not to prevent or treat scoliosis.

After you identify the   abnormal curve you have to identify the cause of the abnormal curve and

have a program in place to remove
the cause and   with spinal
exercises, swimming and the
monkey bar to stop the progression
of scoliosis curve.

If you do nothing and you just wait
and see the scoliosis will get worse,
no matter if you have the
screening for scoliosis in school
by doing the Adams test .

You have   to use the Adams test to
identify the abnormal spinal curve ,
and implement the program for
preventing and correcting the
scoliosis with exercises and redo
the test periodically to see if the
treatments are effective.

For the prevention of scoliosis,

 I recommend that all youngsters
age 7 -18 , and   EVEN YOUNGER,
exercise daily, and this is good for
anyone else who wants to have a
strong, healthy and flexible spine
without any abnormal spinal
curves.

**The exercises I recommend are :
from the S.A.F.E. EXERCISES**

1)SPINAL STRETCH WHILE LYING DOWN FACE UP.

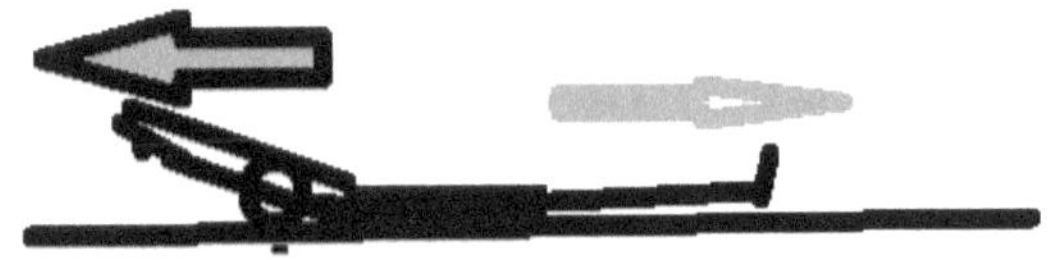

EXTEND YOUR HANDS ABOVE YOUR HEAD TRYING
TO REACH AS FAR AS YOU CAN
AND SIMULTANEOUSLY
 WITH YOUR FEET   TOGETHER TOUCHING THE
MATTRESS STRETCH THEM DOWN AS FAR AS
YOU CAN

THIS IS A SPINAL STRETCH EXERCISE
FEEL THE SPINAL STRETCH

3) SPINAL STRETCH RAISING YOUR HEAD TOWARDS YOUR CHEST

WHILE SUPPORTING YOUR HEAD WITH YOUR HANDS

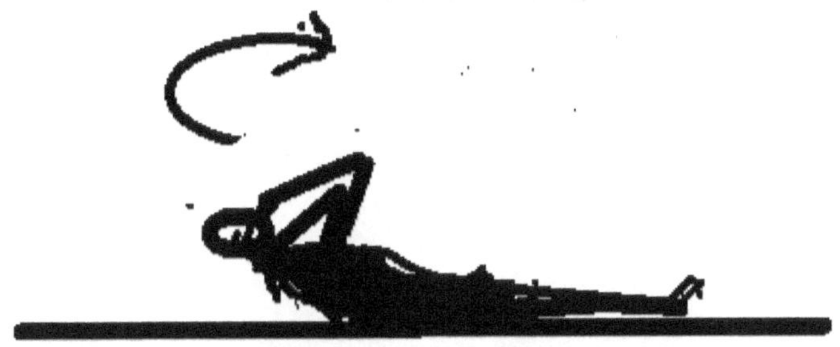

RAISE YOUR HEAD TO YOUR CHEST AS
MUCH AS YOU CAN WITHOUT STRAINING
YOURSELF,
AND THEN LET YOUR HEAD AND HANDS
GENTLY DOWN TO THE MATTRESS.

9) KNEES TO CHEST EXERCISE

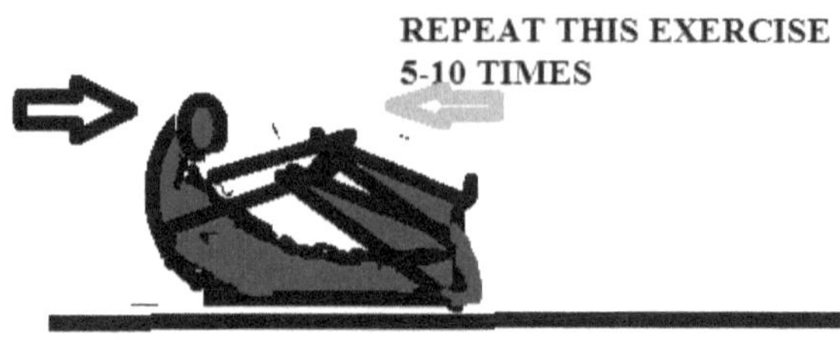

WITH YOUR KNEES BENT DRAW BOTH KNEES TO YOUR CHEST,
GRAB YOUR KNEES WITH BOTH HANDS DRAWING THE KNEES AS NEAR
TO THE CHEST AS POSSIBLE.
AND THEN RAISE YOUR HEAD TOWARDS YOUR KNEES

WITHOUT STRAINING YOURSELF

HOLD IT FOR THE COUNT OF TWO

THEN LOWER YOUR HEAD GENTLY TO THE MATTRESS
AND YOUR FEET TO THE MATTRESS

10)KNEES TO CHEST ROCKING EXERCISE

Knees to chest rocking exercises :

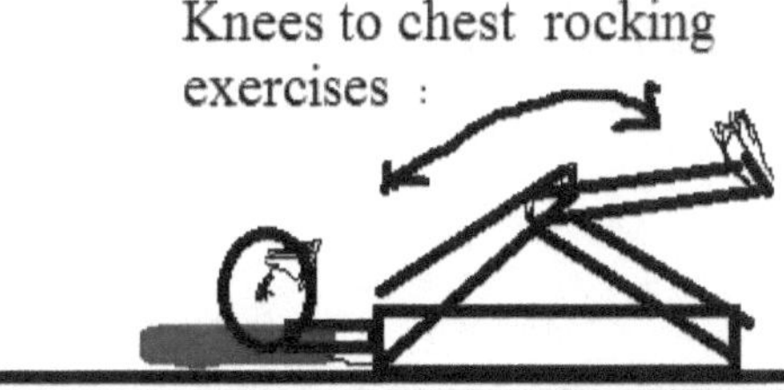

this is the most important exercise to increase the flexibility of your spine.

grab your right knee with your right hand and your left knee with your left hand and bring your knees to your chest and with a rocking motion rock your pelvis back and forth

The modified Adam's forward bend exercise

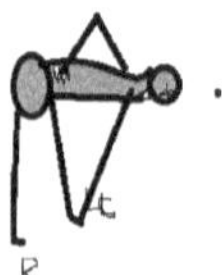

START WITH THE STANDING POSITION BUT
YOUR FEET ARE PLACED 12-18 INCHES APART
BEND FORWARDS AND TOUCH YOUR LEFT
FOOT WITH YOUR RIGHT HAND FINGERS
WHILE YOUR LEFT HAND RESTS ON THE BACK
OF YOUR LOW BACK

The monkey bar exercise

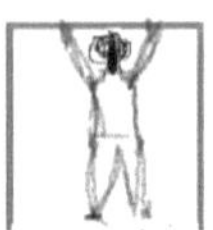

EXERCISING
ON THE
MONKEY BAR

And swimming

**If you have time and do all the
S.A.FE. Exercises every morning
when you wake up that's even
better.**

**Always remember that prevention
is better than trying to   cure it !**

**GET INTO THE HABIT TO   DO THE
EXERCISES WHEN YOU WAKE UP
IN THE MORNING IN YOUR BED
BEFORE YOU GET UP.**

CHAPTER FOURTEEN

THINGS TO DO THAT ARE GOOD FOR THE SPINE

1) ALWAYS SIT STRAIGHT WHEN YOU READ, WORK ON THE COMPUTER, IN CLASS AT SCHOOL AND ESPECIALLY WHEN YOU WATCH TV OR MOVIES............

NEVER SLOUCH ON THE SOFA

2) DO GET UP AND MOVE AROUND
OFTEN,
 STANDING OR SITTING TOO LONG
STRESSES   THE SPINE

 3) PLAY SPORTS, SWIMMING,
SOCCER, And VOLLEY BALL BUT
DO NOT OVERDO IT.....!

 4) DANCING IS OK BUT NO DIPS
OR WILD MOVES

DANCING IS GOOD FOR YOUR
MIND AND BODY.

 IT IS A GOOD RELAXING
EXERCISE

 BUT DO NOT OVER DO IT!

5)TRY TO SLEEP ON YOUR BACK IF
NOT TRY TO SWITCH   SIDES
DURING THE NIGHT FROM LEFT
TO RIGHT AND VICE VERSA

CHAPTER FIFTEEN

  THINGS TO AVOID THAT ARE BAD
FOR YOUR SPINE

1) DO NOT SLEEP ON YOUR
STOMACH,
 Although the face down position
WOULD BE very good for relaxing
and even sleep if the mattress
makers made a perfect hole in their
mattresses for the face while lying
face down, like the hole the
massage tables have.
But with the regular mattresses we
have now it is not a good idea to
sleep face down as it put a lot of
twisting pressure on the upper back
and especially on the neck and can

cause scoliosis on the thoracic cervical(neck) area, other health problems, like headaches, neck pain, shoulder and arm pain.

2) DO NOT RUN FOR LONG DISTANCE UNLESS YOU ARE TRAINED AND HAVE THE NECESSARY GEAR, LIKE PROPER RUNNING SHOES.

3) DO NOT PLAY ON THE TRAMPOLINE, YOU CAN HURT YOURSELF ., UNLESS YOU HAVE PROPER TRAINING

4) NO HEAVY LIFTING AND ALWAYS BEND YOUR KNEES WHEN YOU PICK UP SOMETHING EVEN A PEN...

5) DO NOT CARRY HEAVY OBJECTS OR OVERLOADED BACKPACKS........AND NEVER CARRY YOUR BACK   ON ONE SIDE OF YOUR BODY EVEN IF IT IS NOT HEAVY, THIS FORCES YOUR SPINE INTO A SCOLIOTIC CURVE ...

6) AVOID BAD SITTING POSITIONS WHEN YOU READ, WORK ON THE COMPUTER, AT SCHOOL AND ESPECIALLY WHEN YOU WATCH TV OR MOVIES.........

BAD SITTING CAUSES A LOT OF HEALTH PROBLEMS INCLUDING SCOLIOSIS AND OTHER POSTURAL PROBLEMS

7)IF YOU HAVE YOUNGER SIBLINGS OR NIECES AND NEPHEWS DO NO LIFT OR HOLD THEM ON ONE SIDE OF YOUR BODY, AS THIS MIGHT BE THE CAUSE OF SCOLIOSIS..............

 IF YOU BABY-SIT DO NOT LIFT KIDS OR BABIES AND NEVER EVER HOLD BABIES ON ONE SIDE OF YOUR BODY.

 8)NO HORSING AROUND OR PLAYING PRACTICAL JOKES ON OTHERS AND IN RETURN THEY PLAY PRACTICAL JOKES ON YOU, THIS CAN CAUSE INJURIES TO

YOUR SPINE AND CAUSE A
SCOLIOTIC CURVE .

 MANY PEOPLE WERE INJURED
AND HAD CATASTROPHIC
INJURIES FROM HORSING AROUND
AND PRACTICAL JOKES.

 9) AVOID   CONTACT SPORTS LIKE
FOOTBALL, WRESTLING AND
HOCKEY.

The practice of targeting the good
players   of the other team, to
injure them and get them off the
game so that the other team win ,
SHOULD BE OUTLAWED AND
CRIMINALIZED. I was appalled,
shocked and dismayed while
watching hockey on television to
see a player attack the best player
of the opposite team from behind
and driving the head of that payer
on the ice causing him serious
injuries.
That's   AN INTENTIONAL
CRIMINAL assault causing serious
injuries and should be recognized
as such ,outlawed , frowned upon
such acts and   proper punishment

,like jail time and ban from playing
that sport.

 The motto should be ,' may the
best player win fair and square.",
and not "lets injure him so that we
win." Kids that are watching will
try to do it too and that's very
dangerous.!

CHAPTER SIXTEEN

CONCLUSION

Considering the human suffering and the huge amounts of money spend in this preventable disease, the scoliosis,
I hope that the health professionals that first diagnose this condition will advice their patients what to do to avoid the progression of the curve, avoid expensive treatments and risky surgeries,
by giving them a copy of my designed exercises, S.A.F.E.

'what's good for your spine' and

'what to avoid to have a good strong spine."

It is obvious that the status quo ,

'" of wait and see approach", is not working and many youngsters end up using spinal braces and risky surgeries .

 It is also my hope that governments and schools will have an active role in screening for scoliosis and encourage youngsters to exercise more during school hours, like many companies do with their workers providing exercise time during working hours to prevent scoliosis , and provide ergonomic desks and chairs There is no magic pill and never will be any magic pill to correct the spinal curves but with exercises you can keep your spine in good shape and without abnormal curves.

 To have a strong , flexible and healthy spine you have to exercise daily to have strong spinal muscles .

Athletes that exercise daily, like body builders, swimmers runners and others, have strong healthy spines and rarely if ever get any

abnormal spinal curves like
scoliosis.

 THE SPINAL ACTIVE FLEXION
EXERCISES (S.A.F.E.) I DESIGNED
WILL HELP PEOPLE WITH
SCOLIOSIS AND OTHER SPINAL
CURVATURES   TO GET A
FLEXIBLE, STRONGER HEALTHIER
SPINE

AND EVEN IF A FRACTION   OF
THE MILLIONS OF YOUNGSTERS
WITH SCOLIOSIS ARE HELPED
WITH THE OBSERVATION OF
WILLIAMS ADAMS AND MY
DESIGNED EXERCISES, THIS BOOK
WILL ACCOMPLISH ITS PURPOSE:

 TO HELP AS MANY PEOPLE WITH
SCOLIOSIS AS POSSIBLE.

If you or any of your family and
kids is diagnosed with scoliosis
and" told to wait and see," instead
of waiting in anguish what will
happen down the road in six

months or a year , give my S.A.F.E.
exercises a try with the blessing of
your health provider . You have
nothing to loose and at least your
are doing something about it and
don't be surprised if the scoliosis
reverse itself or at least does not
progress .

 Good luck to every one and may
god   bless the exercises you will be
doing and eliminate your spinal
problems !

CHAPTER SEVENTEEN

EPILOGUE

 I never thought that I will be writing this book.
 However the prospect that my designed exercises will help even a fraction of the millions of people that are suffering from SCOLIOSIS, and with the help of KDP   I did it.

 It is my desire and wish that all those who will DO my designed exercises daily will benefit a lot and prove that I did the right thing to design and publish my   SPINAL ACTIVE FLEXION EXERCISES (S.A.F.E.)

It is my hope   that with exercises
and preventative education   on
how youngsters can take good care
of their spines and proper
treatments, will eliminate   this
preventable disease named
SCOLIOSIS.(crooked spine)

My greatest satisfaction will be
when these exercises help people
with scoliosis, to have a strong ,
healthy flexible spine with less
spinal curvatures and have a
healthier life.

THE AUTHOR

S.ELIA

Disclaimer:
This book is for information ONLY
and is not intended to serve as
medical advice. Anyone seeking
specific advice or assistance should
consult his or her doctor . if they
do not like the advice of their
doctor they should seek a second
opinion from another doctor.

REFERENCES:

1) A Dangerous Curve: The Role of History in America's Scoliosis Screening Programs

2) ADAMS TEST

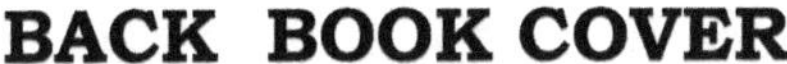
BACK BOOK COVER

SCOLIOSIS:

  A FRESH LOOK AT WHAT
CAUSES THE IDIOPATHIC
FUNCTIONAL SCOLIOSIS AND
HOME EXERCISES TO   STOP THE
PROGRESSION OF THE CURVE
AND EVEN REVERSE IT BACK TO
NORMAL

  HOPE TO EVERY MOTHERS
ANGUISH FOR HER CHILDS
CROOKED SPINE

  TRYING TO TAME THE
ABNORMAL DANGEROUS CURVES
WITH HOME EXERCISES FOR ALL
THOSE WHO ARE DIAGNOSED
WITH SCOLIOSIS, TO STOP THE
PROGRESSION OF THE ABNORMAL
SPINAL CURVE AND GET A
HEALTHY, FLEXIBLE STRONG
SPINE

  Scoliosis is the million dollar
question? How to prevent   it   and
how to stop the progression of the
abnormal spinal curve with home
exercises! And the answer is THE

SPINAL ACTIVE FLEXION. EXERCISES!!(S.A.F.E.)   DONE IN THE PRIVACY OF YOUR HOME IN YOUR OWN BED!

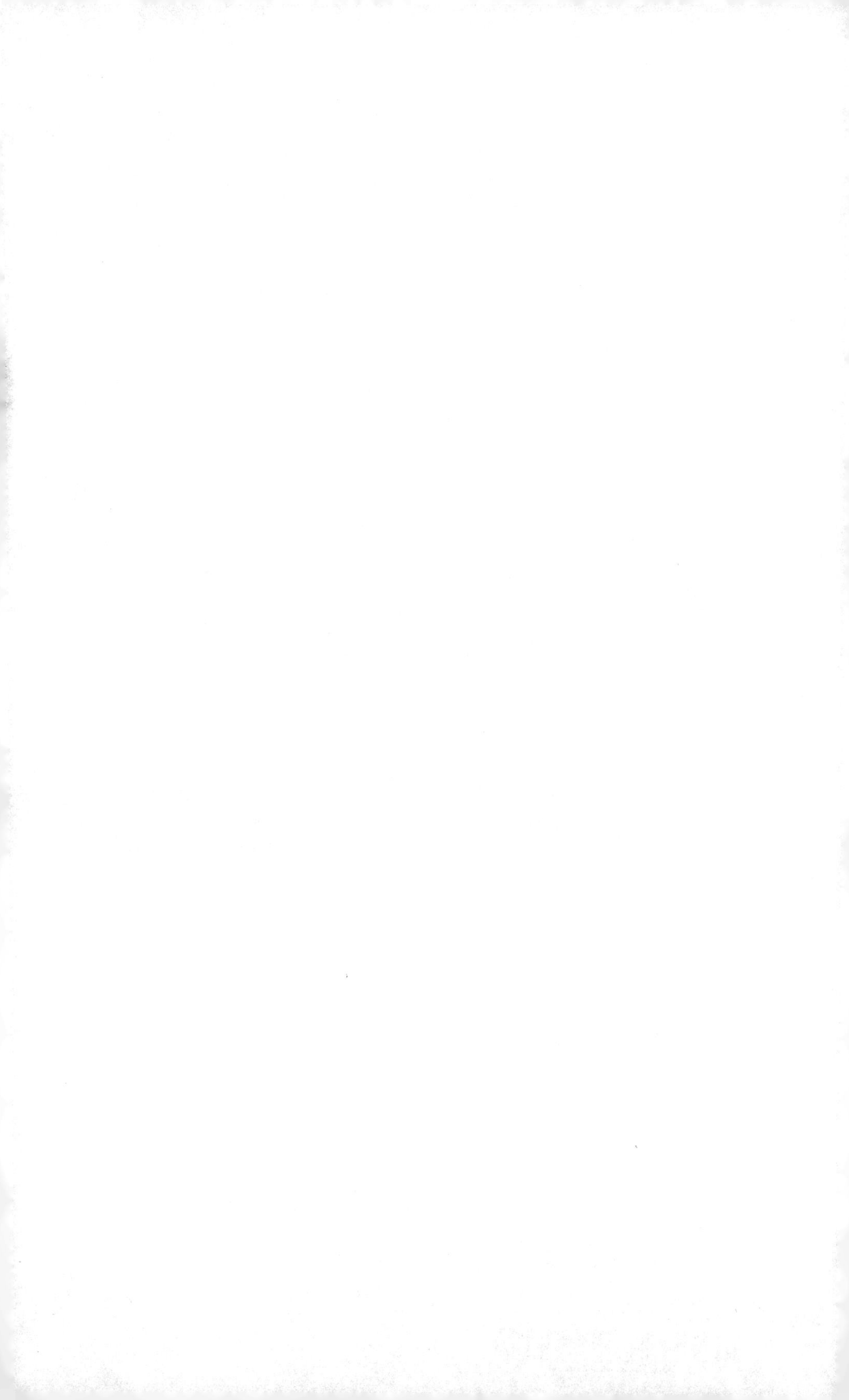

9 781728 674810